Supreme Breath

Yogi Breathing to Access Higher Life Force Energy

Deborah Garland

Forewords by
Shiva Rea
Dr. Swami Shankardev Saraswati

Supreme Breath

Yogi Breathing to Access Higher Life Force Energy

Supreme Breath

Yogi Breathing to Access Higher Life Force Energy

Deborah Garland

Radiance Publishing

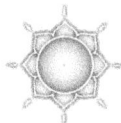

The exercises and practices in this book are not intended to replace the services of your physician, or to provide an alternative to professional medical treatment. *Supreme Breath: Yogi Breathing to Access Higher Life Force Energy* offers no diagnosis of, or treatment, for any specific medical problem that you may have. Where it suggests the possible usefulness of certain practices in relation to certain illnesses or symptoms, it does so solely for educational purposes – either to explore the possible relationship of breathing to health, or to expose the reader to alternative health and healing approaches. The breathing practices outlined here are gentle, and should—if carried out as described— be beneficial to overall physical and psychological health. If you have any serious medical or psychological problems, such as: heart disease, high blood pressure, cancer, mental illness, recent surgeries, or any other medical condition; you should consult your physician before practicing the exercises described here.

Illustrations and Book Design by Deborah Garland

Library of Congress Control Number: 2015910594

ISBN 978-0-692-47566-9

Infinite and Eternal Gratitude to JK

Foreword

In today's busy but mainly sedentary lifestyle, and with an epidemic of chronic illnesses such as heart disease, obesity and cancer increasing, learning how to breathe properly may be the healthiest and most intelligent thing you can do.

In the ancient sciences of yoga, Tai Chi, Chi Gong and in various forms of martial arts, the proper use of the breath, and your ability to tie this to regulation of the heart and the mind is the key to increasing health, vitality and inner power.

When we sit for long hours our muscles become tight and our ability to draw oxygen into the lungs and blood is diminished. We starve ourselves of the most essential life giving substance, which is air. Modern research has called sitting the new smoking. The longer you sit the greater is your chance of degenerative disease.

Medical science is telling us that we have to get up every half and hour and move and breathe for just a few minutes to improve the circulation of the blood, and to feed and nourish our inner organs, such as our brain, heart, liver, pancreas and so on. We neglect ourselves at our own peril.

Eastern traditions see air as being full of subtle force called prāna, vital life energy. This energy can be felt through various yoga-breathing exercises, called pranayama, and through various forms of meditation. The process of attuning oneself to this wonderful life force takes time but the result is worth the effort. You can overcome many forms of illness, feel incredibly vital, and live full of strength and energy at any age. You can have the energy to live a full and meaningful life, and to have an energetic and mobile old age.

In my medical and yoga therapy practice I have been teaching yogic breathing and meditation to thousands of patients over the last 45 years, often combined with appropriate medical and therapeutic interventions with great success. Everyone who practices under guidance derives some form of benefit, be it relaxation, mental calm, a sense of greater energy and wellbeing, and greater resilience in the fight against illness.

Deborah has done a wonderful job to bring together the theory and practice of yogi breathing. If you follow the exercises in this book I am sure you will gain a lot of benefits. Start simply and work your way slowly and progressively through the chapters, exploring what your body and mind need and want and enjoy the process. You only need a little bit of practice to gain a lot of benefits.

Wishing you all peace and good health,
Dr. Swami Shankardev Saraswati
www.bigshakti.com

Foreword

$\mathbf{P}$rana is the source of life.

All beings in every moment are expressions of the primary pulse of life.
Our breath – our rhythm of being alive, spiritus, inspiration, prana- is the tidal flow of our life-force. Inhale – exhale. Receiving – giving. Inward and outward dance of oxygen balancing CO_2.

We seek to breathe – the vital force we cannot exist without – and in so we open to a life-giving force that breathes through us. No one knows the source of breath. Within our often shallow and forgotten breath is a deeper mystery - the breath within the breath - our supreme breath - a source rhythm breathing us all.

Deborah Garland's "*Supreme Breath*" is an accessible and profound guide to the power of breath potential contained in each moment. As a long time yoga practitioner, teacher, mother and global explorer, she bridges the roots of yoga with the universal needs of these pressing times. Conscious breathing or pranayama within yoga and meditation have scientifically proven benefits in transforming stress and enhancing our highest states of flow that positively increase our health and well-being.

Now more than ever, we need to access the healing potential of conscious breathing. We are poisoning the air we breathe, disturbing our rainforest lungs in the face of climate change as unprecedented levels of stress rise. Realizing our breath is of supreme importance to our vital health, balance, longevity and quality of life.

Our breath is our highest pilgrimage available to be experienced 21,600 times a day.

May we awaken to the power of our breath - like solar, wind, and water - renewable sources of untapped energy, ready to be accessed here and now.

Shiva Rea
Delphi, Greece
www.pranavinyasaflow.com

Contents

Introduction

We all dwell within a substratum of universal prana—the natural force that keeps the stars, planets, and galaxies in perpetual motion. Ancient yogis studied and understood the nature of universal prana, and developed sophisticated systems and practices to help human beings live in divine harmony with the natural flow of organic, cosmic energies. We also live in a world with vast amounts of energetic force generated by inorganic technologies. Our energetic field is saturated with invisible signals from satellites, cell phones, and wireless products. Electric currents permeate our living and workspaces, and we are addicted to the stimulating light and sound pulsations from our computers, televisions, and ever-evolving array of digital devices. We are attracted by the strong charges emitted from these inorganic energies. They can pull our awareness away from rhythms of the natural, living pranas that keep our heart beating and our lungs operating.

Imagine how you feel as you stand near a waterfall, pause at the highest peak of a snowy mountain ski slope, enjoy a slow walk through a beautiful flower garden, sit near warm and gentle ocean waves, or smell clean air after a rainstorm. In these experiences you feel a high quantum of prana as your senses absorb natural life force energies into your body, mind, and spirit. Your vital energies become heightened, and you feel more alive, refreshed, and revitalized.

The practice of pranayama, conscious yogi breathing, helps us access heightened life force energies. We don't need to move to a mountaintop or seaside to access this pranic force. It exists everywhere. Through conscious awareness and focused breathing techniques we can create more prana, build pranic reserves, and learn to keep our prana from depleting. We can learn to access higher pranic energies to create abundance, vibrancy, and radiant health in life.

The practice of pranayama provides a platform for awakening a profound understanding of mental, intellectual, and spiritual aspects of ourselves and of our world. Prana is universal in nature. Our individual prana is a microcosm of vast, and unfathomable, universal energy. As awareness of our pranic energy grows, we naturally access subtler facets of our being. We experience greater clarity and insightfulness as our ability to tap into our higher pranic energy evolves. We develop greater discernment and expanded perception. We may come to view and understand certain aspects of our own personal lives and the larger world from a higher vantage point.

A certain amount, or quantum, of prana exists in every person. Prana flows within the physical body through a vast network of energetic channels called nadis to maintain our bones, muscles, tissues, blood, and organs that our body needs to survive. When there is a healthy quantum of prana, and the distribution network of nadis is open and robust, prana can be efficiently distributed to every cell and atom to keep the physical body in good condition.

Pranayama practice can actually create a greater quantum of prana, and expand pranic energy beyond the physical body to the mind, emotional, intellectual, and spiritual parts of ourselves. Just as an efficient flow of prana fuels our physical body to become stronger, healthier, and more available to help navigate us through life; it can also strengthen our mind, emotions, intellect, and spirit.

Through the practice of pranayama, great awakenings of universal pranic energies within us can occur. It is important to practice pranayama with patience and intelligence so that pranic energies are accessed gradually. Too much energy transmitted too soon can be harmful. Imagine trying to send broadband signals into a transistor radio. You certainly would not receive any sound if you tried to turn the radio on, because the transistor technology is not able to handle the signal. If you've ever tried to run the air conditioner, washer, dishwasher, and hair dryer at the same time, you may have tripped a circuit. In this case, the circuitry may be in place and in good working condition, but cannot operate when overloaded with too much energy. Pranayama sends powerful life energy through our system. It's important to practice with patience, gentleness, and mindfulness.

Pranayama can help us increase prana, and also help us conserve, regulate, and store our pranic energy. Everything in life requires prana. Prana is consumed in every conscious and unconscious activity you are involved in, day and night. You might imagine that we all have individual pranic bank accounts, and we can make withdraws and deposits through our thoughts and actions. Just as conscious, healthy lifestyle choices increase and maintain prana, we waste precious pranic energy through anxiety, worries and fears. Pranayama practice can help us create balance and harmony throughout the body, mind, emotions, intellect, and spirit. When pranic energies are strong and regulated, we can build up a healthy pranic reserve to draw upon during turbulent times in life. When we learn to budget our prana, we ensure that our vital pranas remain available to keep our entire human organism functioning at optimal levels at all times.

Our physical, mental, emotional, and spiritual health is dependent on receiving a balanced supply of prana. With increased practice of pranayama we can learn to manipulate the flow of pranic energy in our body. We can supply prana to the specific areas where there is a deficiency, and balance out excess build-up in other areas. Wherever the body feels weak or sick, there is a deficiency of prana. You can help the body heal by learning to supply more prana to those places in the body.

When I was a kid, I developed asthma. I remember lying listlessly on my mother's sofa day upon day, feeling my vital life energies slowly and steadily slipping away from me. I was ten years old and I had forgotten how to breathe. I know now that I coped with an uneasy childhood by holding a great deal of stress in my young body. I tried to buffer myself from the uncertainty of daily life by remaining on guard at all times. I must have kept myself locked into the adrenaline-pumping mode of the "fight or flight" response for long stretches at a time. Holding on to stress in this way keeps the sympathetic nervous system activated, never allowing the relaxing, soothing effects of the parasympathetic nervous system to kick into gear and bathe the body and mind with vital pranic energy. It's a common response to stress.

I'm pretty sure I chronically tightened my respiratory diaphragm and, over time, developed a habit of shallow breathing. My lungs became severely depleted of prana. My respiratory system became weak and inefficient. Eventually, anytime something went awry at home and I felt unsafe, there I went into the dreaded asthma attack. It was an awful cycle.

I was not taught about prana as a child, but fortunately I came into this world as a naturally curious and spiritual kid. I intently observed the behaviors of people, places, and things around me with a driving determination to understand how all the pieces fit together in the world. I took great comfort in nature. In the amazing world of bugs, fish, flowers, trees, sunsets, and thunderstorms; I felt I could breathe. Outside in nature, my young, depleted lungs soaked up the natural energies of universal life force as I saw, smelled, touched, heard, and tasted the vibrant pulsations of pure prana, prana shakti. Even though as a child I could not explain why or how, I knew that my body, mind, and spirit felt more alive, stronger, and stable when I immersed myself in these higher, natural pranas.

As I learned to access and draw in greater pranic energy, my need for the constant company of the albuterol inhaler gradually diminished. I have not experienced an asthmatic episode in nearly forty years. The study, practice, and teaching of yoga and pranayama continue to open my awareness to higher pranas and deeper insights. I feel extremely fortunate to have studied with true master teachers very early in my exploration of yoga and pranayama. I am deeply and infinitely grateful to Shiva Rea and Swami Shankardev Saraswati who so generously and masterfully laid solid groundwork, and brilliantly illuminated my path. I feel tremendously honored to have studied with luminaries Dr. Vasant Lad, Dr. David Frawley (Pandit Vamadeva Shastri), Dr. Robert Svoboda, Erich Schiffmann, Gurmukh Khalsa, Hari Jap, Rama Jyoti Vernon, and Bhavani Maki.

The practices in this book are pure, authentic techniques, originating from ancient Vedic teachings and long-held yogic lineages. The advanced knowledge of ancient rishis and sages evolved well before the technological era. We do not live in a culture with constant awareness of the flow of organic cycles and seasons of earth, sun, stars, and planets as they did; but these organic rhythms are what our cells, tissues, muscles bones, and souls understand. The information and exercises in this book have been known by yogis for thousands of years to slow and reverse the effects of aging, reduce stress, achieve optimal health, and access your highest inner source of eternal radiance… your own vital life force energy, your prana.

You will discover authentic yogic pranayamas and find simple, uplifting, and easy to follow methods to develop a deeper awareness of your physical, mental, intellectual, and emotional layers, bringing them into perfect harmony. You will discover how to use breathing to feel balanced, healthy, and youthful. You will learn to handle the ups and downs of life with grace and ease, soon shining with a luminous glow from within. Mastering yogi breathing techniques will allow you to embrace life with a whole new vibrant awareness, and gain access to your highest life force energies.

Thank you for being here!

Supreme Breath
Yogi Breathing to Access Higher Life Force Energy

Begin.
Begin this very moment.
Breathe.
Breathe In.
Breathe Out.
Begin Again.

*T*his is a very simple book. It's a simple book with simple techniques for doing something you continuously do each and every day and each and every night of your life - breathing.

Breathing is simple and instinctual, and most of us have forgotten how to do it. Have you ever seen a little baby breathe? As breath comes in, the little baby's entire body seems to inflate. With each gentle breath every bone, muscle, tissue, and cell pulsates with pure, peaceful, vibrant life source. The yogis call this vital energy prana. Natural, relaxed, deep breathing fills us with prana.

Over time we develop habits and patterns of thoughts and behaviors, keeping us stuck in repetitive swirls of emotions, stresses, and tensions that constrict and obstruct the flow of prana. As a result, our breath becomes shallow, irregular, quick, choppy, and thin. As our breath weakens, our natural, vital life force diminishes. But when our breath is robust, our vital life force is vibrant. Our breath carries prana and distributes it throughout the body. This vital energy keeps us alive. Breath is life, and life is breath.

Right now, observe the way you are breathing. Pause for a few moments and pay attention to your breath. Don't try to change anything, just observe. How closely do you feel your breathing pattern resembles the way you breathed as a little baby – full, natural, relaxed, and peaceful? Close your eyes for a few moments and imagine yourself breathing in the way a baby breathes. Your breath flows smoothly, deeply, evenly, and fully. Your back and ribs and chest and belly soften and inflate easily as your breath comes in. Your whole body relaxes as the breath flows out. Really imagine it and experience it. After only a few moments breathing in this natural way, notice how you feel.

Focusing awareness on your breath has a calming effect on the mind. As you become aware of your breath, your mind becomes tranquil. As your mind becomes calm, your body relaxes, and tension blockages are released. As you relax, your vital energy flows and pulsates rhythmically throughout all the layers and systems of your body to nourish you, heal you, and revitalize you.

The yogis mastered the art of breathing. They understood that breath is both the physical act of respiration and the act of distributing prana. Prana is our vital life force and a powerful healing energy in the body that can optimize our physical, mental, emotional, and spiritual wellbeing.

In this book, we explore the very natural and profound practice of pranayama—yogi breathing. There is much to remember, but not so much to learn, because you were born knowing how

Begin

Your first breath begins at birth, and your last breath at death. Fully celebrate and embrace the beautiful magnificence of each breath in between.

Introduction

Deep

Breathe deep.
Slow and deep.
Avoid quick and
shallow. Dive in
deep.

to breathe. You were born breathing organically, synchronized in perfect harmony with the rhythms and pulsations of nature, of universal prana. You were born knowing how to balance and direct your vital life force to maintain radiant health, inexhaustible energy, and immense happiness in this life.

Let's begin. Begin to draw in. Begin to let go. Explore, expand, renew. Revitalize, remember, understand. Begin to breathe.

Easy Slow Breath

Slow down your breathing. Close your eyes. Fill your lungs as slowly, deeply, and evenly as you can. When you feel that your lungs are completely full, expand and bring in just a little bit more air. Slowly, gently and smoothly let your breath flow out. Feel your lungs deflate. Do it again and again. Keep your throat soft as you transition from inhale to exhale. Slow down some more until you feel ease and relaxation.

You Already Know How to Breathe

You can rest assured that your body knows how to breathe. Sometimes we make our lives more challenging by relying too much on our mind to "figure it out" or "do it the right way." When you are truly relaxed in your natural state, your breath and prana flow harmoniously all on their own.

Try this... lie down or sit comfortably. Relax. Breathe in and wait. Do nothing and wait. In time your body will exhale by its own nature. After you exhale, wait. Do nothing. Relax and wait. Do nothing at all. Just wait. Your body will inhale.

Continue the process. Inhale, relax, be still, do nothing, and wait. Do nothing. Exhalation will naturally happen. Then relax, be still, do nothing, and wait. Relax, be patient, and wait. Breath will flow in. The pattern repeats over and over and over again.

Mindful

Pranayama is mindfulness.

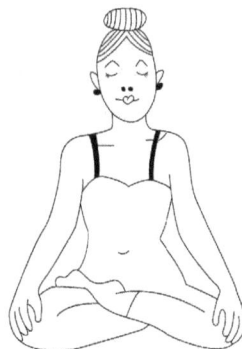

Relaxed Posture

How to Use This Book

Pranayama is for everyone, and there is a little something in this book for everyone. If you are a health care practitioner, teacher, student, business executive, mom, dad, spiritual seeker, or experiencing your unique expression as a fellow human on this beautiful path of life, there is something in this book for you. No matter if you are learning diaphragmatic breathing to recover from an illness, studying pranayama techniques to teach in your yoga class or school, or simply looking to elevate the quality of your life and those you love, the techniques in this book will help you.

I encourage everyone to begin by reading the introductory information about prana. It's important to establish a framework and foundational understanding about the nature of prana and how we can manipulate our vital life force energy with our conscious awareness and breath. At first you may not grasp the Sanskrit

Introduction

Receive

Be still and very, very patient. Be soft and quiet and still. Allow perfect waves of beautiful breath flow deeply into you.

words, but that's perfectly okay. Wherever possible, I include common, everyday descriptions of Vedic concepts and words. If you would like to use the Sanskrit words (and I sincerely hope that you do) there is a glossary with pronunciations and definitions of key terms.

It's important to master the essential pranayamas. Not necessarily all of the essential pranayamas, but do not proceed without mastering breath awareness, diaphragmatic breathing, and ujjayi. There are lots of breathing practices and techniques presented here. I need to emphasize that mastery is the goal, not variety. Yogis spend years—even lifetimes—on just one breath technique. It's best to practice a technique, or level of practice, for weeks before moving on. Subtleties in your practice will begin to emerge over time that will yield vast benefits and rewards. Go slowly, patiently, and gently. Try to stick with a practice and truly delve into it. Even if you are curious and want to try several exercises, don't abandon committed, long-term exploration of a chosen technique.

When you practice a technique, use the Goldilocks approach: not too fast, not too slow, but just right; not too forceful, not too weak, but just right. Practice with gentleness, moderation, and keen awareness at all times. It is important to practice with discernment. If something does not resonate with you, or doesn't feel quite right, then do not engage in the practice. Allow your inner wisdom to guide you.

Try to keep a pen or pencil handy when you pick up this book. There is ample blank space for you to write about your thoughts, reactions, experiences, and insights. Take time to pause and fully experience the breathing exercises and meditations, then describe your experiences. Revisit them and note how your experiences and insights evolve and shift over time.

*Follow these general guidelines when practicing pranayama.
If you have a physical or mental health condition that may be of
concern, check with your health care provider before practicing any
pranayama techniques.*

Real

*Breath is real
life. Life is real
breath. Really
breathe, really
live.*

* NEVER STRAIN in any way.
* Practice with a gentle, smooth, and steady breath.
* Stop at any sign of fatigue or discomfort.
* Practice on an empty stomach.
* Less is more, avoid extreme effort.
* Warm up the physical body with yoga asana before pranayama.
* Always breathe through the nose, unless instructed otherwise.
* Keep the spine straight and body relaxed.
* Stay with simple, calming pranayamas for a good while, perfecting the technique and feeling the effects before moving on to additional practices.
* Focus on the subtle energy layers more than the physical body.
* Accept and understand that pranayama requires time, patience, practice, and perseverance.
* Some side effects of pranayama in healthy individuals may be sensations of tingling in the skin, feelings of heat, cold, lightness, or heaviness. This is normal and is part of the process of purification and releasing toxins from the system. If symptoms persist, medical advice is suggested.
* If dizziness or nausea is experienced during pranayama, stop the practice, lie down, and relax. If discomfort persists do not continue the practice until medical advice is obtained.
* Never practice if taking drugs or alcohol.
* Never practice breath retention, bhastrika, or kapalbhati if heart conditions, glaucoma, hernia, ulcers, stroke, epilepsy, vertigo, or high blood pressure are present.
* When in doubt, seek medical advice.
* NEVER, EVER FORCE OR STRAIN IN ANY WAY.
* Above all, truly enjoy your pranayama!!

Introduction

Prana:
Vital Life Force Energy

Vital life force energy is known by many names in eastern philosophies, martial arts, and in western sciences as: chi, ki, qi, energy, and prana. Ancient seers recognized the power of universal, multidimensional life force energy, which is found throughout the cosmos called mahaprana, or the greatest prana. This universal energy forms the foundation for all of life. Swami Sivananda Saraswati described prana as the sum total of all energy that is manifest in the universe and the sum total of all the forces of nature. All the forms of energy we know, heat, light, electricity and magnetism are forms of prana. Everything in our world that you observe or sense is an expression of prana.

In Vedic philosophy, human life is a microcosm of a greater macrocosm. We hear the words, "as above so below," and understand that the forces responsible for maintaining the workings of the entire cosmos, our universe and solar system, are also the same forces responsible for maintaining our individual lives. All life on earth is dependent on the vital, heating and life-supporting energy radiating from the sun. As we look around our environment, we see plants, animals, and humans all energized by solar prana shakti—the natural force of pure energy supporting all life on our planet. Prana shakti is a very powerful energy, and it exists within all matter.

The practices of yoga and pranayama seek to tap into the force of prana shakti by unlocking dormant energy stored in the base of the spine. This dormant energy is known as kundalini shakti. As the sleeping kundalini shakti activates, it begins to rise up higher and higher through the center of the spine from the base to the head, and we are able to access vast amounts of pure and powerful pranic energy.

Nourish

Our breath is the physical, gross breath, and also the very subtle life force, prana.

We can consider these vital life force energies as stored pure potential, unlimited possibilities, and infinite opportunities just waiting to be tapped into. We may have experienced fleeting awareness of our prana shakti energy potential during an "ah ha" moment, a feeling of indescribable joy, or a wave of powerful or creative strength that seemed to appear from out of the blue. But this awareness does not need to be a random or an unpredictable occurrence. We can use pranayama, conscious yogi breathing, to thoughtfully access and utilize our higher life force, our higher pranic energies in all areas of our lives.

What is Prana?

Prana is our vital essence – our life force. When prana is present, there is life. When prana leaves, there is death. In the Sanskrit language, *pra* may be translated as constant, and *na* as movement. Prana can be considered vital, universal energy that is constantly in motion. Breath is the vehicle, the carrier of prana in our body. When we stop breathing, prana ceases to flow, and our life stops.

Prana is the vital life force responsible for our physical, mental, emotional, and spiritual existence. Prana is the vital energy that permeates each and every cell and atom in our body. When our

*High pranas
are present
at all times.
Simply awaken
your sensory
perception of
them.*

prana is balanced and robust we feel good. We feel strong, nourished, and happy. We radiate, glowing with health and youthful vibrancy. We feel lighthearted, with a spring in our step and sparkle in our eyes.

When our prana is depleted, or imbalanced, we feel weak, stressed, run down, and unhealthy. We feel sluggish, lethargic, confused, and may feel as if the simplest of tasks require tremendous effort. We feel as if we're continually running on a low battery.

Prana is subtle and immensely powerful. Prana is like a refined, precious, transparent current of magnetic energy supplying living, renewable vitality. We all experience prana, yet it is elusive and difficult to characterize. Prana is ethereal and multidimensional. In our daily lives we may be aware of how we are feeling, we discern symptoms and sensations in various parts of our bodies, and we perceive diversified states of our emotions. Fluctuations in our physical, mental, and emotional conditions reflect the changeable qualities of prana.

Without prana we could not function as human beings. But our bodies can lose prana with environmental, emotional, and physical stress. Everyday tensions, worries and anxieties deplete prana. Overloading the senses with too much external stimuli such as: computers, TV, smart phones, and gaming devices depletes prana. Generally too much doing, too much thinking, too much external activity of all sorts, can drain our prana. If we allow our prana to weaken, dissipate, and generally run low, our body degenerates and disease processes may begin.

If we balance, preserve, and maximize our prana, our vital life force energy flows freely, permeating our entire being, and enhancing the quality of our lives. We retain our health and vitality as we age. We naturally detoxify our body. Our cells are nourished and rejuvenated. Our skin is supple and beautifully radiant. We have more energy and reduced stress. Our eyes sparkle and shine. We feel happier, look younger, and we are more vibrantly alive.

Life

There is a famous story about Prana found in ancient Vedic teachings. As told in the Chandogya Upanishad, the main senses were arguing with each other about which of them was most important to life. To settle their argument, they decided that, one by one, each would leave the body and see how the body got along without it.

First speech departed, but the body continued to survive. Next eyesight left, but the body continued in spite of blindness. Next, hearing departed, but the body continued. The sense of smell left, but the body continued without the ability to smell. The mind left, but the body continued to live without consciousness. Finally, Prana began to leave, but the body began to die. All the senses began to follow prana, just as honey bees follow the queen as she leaves the hive.

So all the senses begged Prana to remain in the body. It was settled. The senses declared Prana the most supreme and vital for life. With Prana there is life, without Prana there can be no life

---

We Feel Prana Differently in Each Area of Our Body

Our pranic energy flows through our physical body primarily through the respiratory and circulatory systems. Prana takes on unique qualities in different parts of our bodies. For example, we

*Where
Awareness Goes,
Energy Flows.*

feel heavier and denser in the lower parts of our body, and lighter in the upper parts. As we begin to develop a greater awareness of our own prana, we naturally begin to finely tune our sensory perceptions of our vital energy. We learn tune into our bodies and develop an ability to feel when prana becomes weak, blocked, or sluggish. We learn to take action to restore a vital, healthy pranic flow before degeneration or disease processes can begin. There are five predominate directional movements of vital life force energies within the body called pancha vayus (PAHN-chah) (VAH-EE-oo).

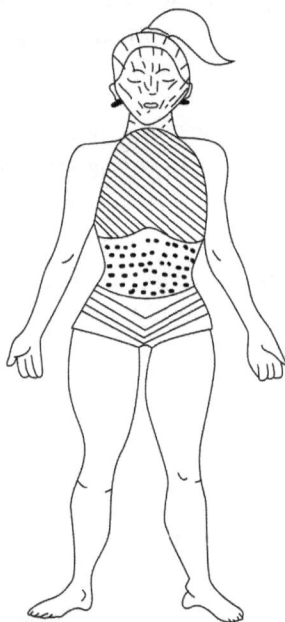

udana

prana

samana

apana

uyana
(throughout body)

Pancha Vayus

Heavy, dense, and downward moving prana is concentrated in the pelvic area, from the navel to the perineum. This prana is called apana vayu and is associated with elimination and reproduction.

Prana drawing inward from the periphery of the body to the center is called samana. It is concentrated in the midsection, circulates around the navel, and governs digestion and assimilation.

Prana located in the chest area is also called prana. It is responsible for breathing and bringing fresh energy into the body. Prana draws breath inward. We feel our lungs and chest inflate, and experience the force of prana from the navel to the throat as light, upward moving, and expansive.

Udana is light, upward moving prana from the throat to the head. Udana can also be experienced as spiraling energy through the arms and legs ascending upward toward the head.

Vyana is prana that permeates every cell in the entire body. Vyana supports all the other pranas and moves in all directions. It can be felt as vital energy in the heart region, radiating outward from the center to the periphery, and beyond the boundaries of the skin.

While all of the vayus are important in the practice of pranayama, many breathing techniques aim to consciously manipulate the flow of apana and prana. Some yogis consider prana and apana the most important vayus in the body. Prana is responsible for bringing energy into the body through respiration, and apana is responsible for moving energies, toxins, and wastes through the openings in the lower part of the body. Vital health requires prana and apana to be in balance. In pranayama practice, we pull apana up and bring prana down to become assimilated in samana at the navel center. The pranic fields merge with one another and are distributed throughout the body, mind, and subtle energy layers

Flow

Prana organically flows in divine harmony with the entire cosmos.

Prana: Vital Life Force Energy

Pulsate

Be very still and feel your vital energy pulsate in perfect, divine harmony with the rhythms of the universe.

helping to balance all the pranas. Vital life force energy is infused into every cell and atom, resulting in vibrancy, radiance, and the highest quality of life experience on every level.

. . .

The importance of developing awareness of the five vayus cannot be underestimated. Knowing how pranas feel within the body really helps you tune into the changing nature of pranic flow. You can feel and make subtle corrections as imbalances arise. When you develop an intimate understanding of how healthy pranic flow feels in your body, you will naturally feel it when energies begin get out of balance. You will feel as if something is not quite right. But with greater awareness, you can learn to tune into the area of the body where imbalance is occurring.

For example, I teach group yoga classes early in the morning. Often during 6am class, students struggle with standing balance poses, like tree and dancing warrior, where you stand on one leg. Steadiness in balance poses requires strong apana vayu—down-ward moving energy. Imbalance in these poses can usually be corrected by sending awareness to the seat of apana vayu—the area from the navel to the pelvic floor, building strength there, then sending the awareness down the legs to the feet. Weak apana, especially early in the morning, can also indicate holding on to emotional energies that have accumulated during sleep. Weak apana can also indicate inadequate elimination of the bowels, or constipation. Strong, energizing pranayamas can help circulate vital prana, releasing emotional and physical stagnation.

Prana Flows through Channels and Energy Centers

Prana can be described as multi-dimensional energy in constant motion. Our prana flows in currents, or pathways, similar to the flow of ocean currents, rivers, radio waves, or electromagnetic currents. Prana moves through our physical and subtle energy body within a vast network of pathways called nadis (NAH-dee). Some nadi channels are very large, carrying a large quantum of prana, while others are miniscule. Ancient yogic texts identify thousands of these pathways. Some texts refer to 72,000 and upwards of 350,000 nadis.

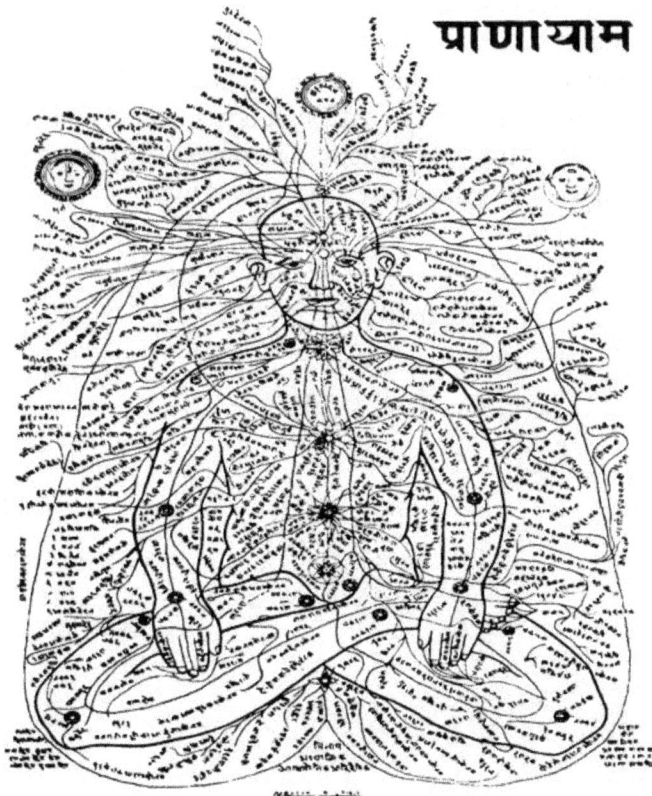

प्राणायाम

Tune

Finely tune your awareness to feel the magnificent power of prana shakti - pure vital energy.

Prana moves through the nadis, supplying vital energy to each and every cell and atom in our bodies. Nadis also carry very subtle pranic energies, enabling us to experience emotional, mental, and spiritual awareness. When prana flows freely through this network of nadis, we are nourished, enlivened, and vibrantly healthy – physically, emotionally, and spiritually. But when the nadi channels become congested, blocked, or unbalanced, the flow of prana is disturbed and our overall health and well-being diminishes. We may become physically ill, emotionally unsteady, and feel a general sense of unease.

Of the thousands of nadis, the most important are three primary channels called ida (EE-duh), pingala (PEEN-gah-luh), and sushumna (soo-SHOOM-nuh). Ida nadi is cooling, soothing, and feminine in nature. It is associated with mental energy and the parasympathetic nervous system. Pingala nadi is stimulating, heating, and masculine in nature. It is associated with active pranic energy and the sympathetic nervous system. Sushumna nadi is the main, central channel, associated with robust vitality and spiritual energy.

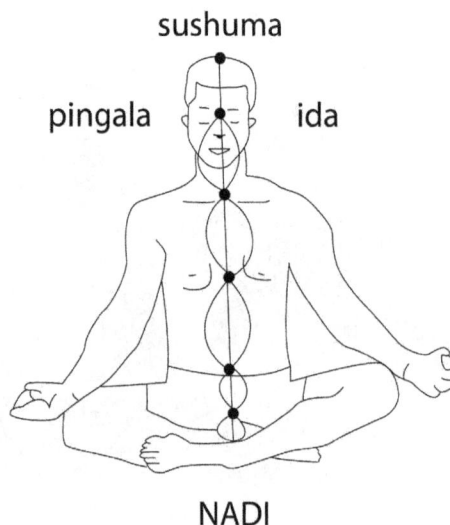

sushuma

pingala   ida

NADI

All three nadis originate near the base of the spine. The sushumna travels up the center of the spine and to the crown of the head. Ida rises upward from the left, and pingala from the right, and spirals around the sushumna to meet at the center of the eyebrows. As they coil around the central channel, ida and pingala intersect the sushumna in six places: the base of the spine, top of pubic bone, navel, heart, throat, and eyebrow center. Ida then flows through the left nostril, and pingala flows through the right.

We see the balanced flow of prana depicted in the ancient symbol associated with medicine and healing, as the caduceus. The central staff in the caduceus correlates with the spinal channel, the sushumna. The twisted snakes represent the ida and pingala channels. When these channels are unobstructed and flowing freely with prana, vital health is present.

The intersections where ida and pingala meet are confluences of concentrated pranic energy called chakras (CHAH-krah). Thousands of nadis flow from each chakra center, distributing prana to every part of the body.

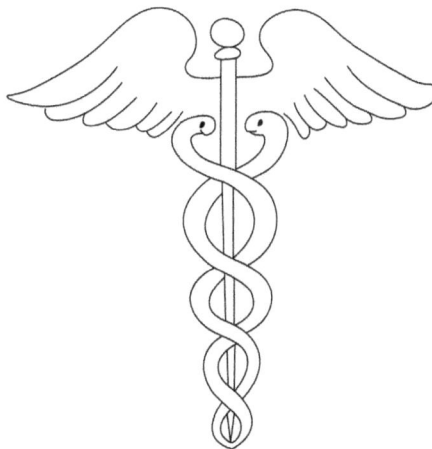

Prana is distributed through the base chakra, muladhara (MOO-lah-dhah-ruh), providing energy for elimination and

Caduceus

establishing an emotional sense of security and foundation. The second chakra, swadhisthana (swah-dhi-STAH-nuh), supplies prana to the genitourinary system and our sense of creativity and sexuality. The navel center, manipura (mah-nee-POOR-ruh), supplies prana to the digestive system and our feelings of strength and willpower.

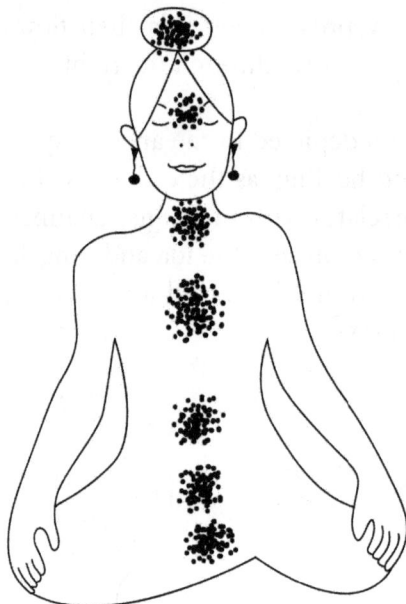

sahasrara

ajna

vishuddhi

anahata

manipura

swadhisthana

manipura

Chakras

Anahata (ah-NAH-hah-tuh), the heart chakra, supplies prana to the respiratory and cardiovascular systems, and is responsible for our feelings of love and compassion. The throat center, vishuddhi (vih-SHOO-dhuh), distributes prana to the sensory organs in our head, and our sense of self-expression through speech. Ajna (AHGN-yah) chakra, in the center of the forehead, supplies prana to our brain and supplies pranic energy for our insights and intuitive awareness. The sushumna rises higher to pierce the crown chakra, sahasrara (sah-hah-SRAH-ruh) where supreme pranic energy illuminates our highest consciousness.

Learning to feel the flow of prana through the right and left channels, the pingala and ida nadis, can help you maintain balance and focus throughout the day. The pingala nadi carries vital prana shakti energy, and the ida nadi carries mental prana, chitta energy. Simply by being aware of breath smoothly flowing in and out of the nostrils, you are helping balance your physical and mental energies.

Love

Yes, truly, all you need is LOVE. Feel love, breathe love.

Take a moment to feel the flow of breath through the nostrils. Does one nostril feel more open, with a stronger flow of prana? Throughout the day, the ida and pingala switch dominance. Pingala will be stronger for about two hours, then ida becomes stronger. When the right nostril is flowing stronger, your digestion and physical strength is higher. When the left nostril is flowing stronger, your body is ready to slow down and relax.

. . .

Here is a yogi weight management tip. Eat meals when the right nostril is flowing strongly. This is when your metabolism is efficient and digestive fire is high. If it is mealtime and your left nostril is flowing, you can change the dominance to make pingala nadi stronger. Simply sit quietly and press your right hand into your left armpit. Hold it there, breathing slowly for five minutes, or until the right nostril begins to flow... then enjoy your meal!

Koshas: Sheaths of Energy Frequency

Each human being is comprised of energetic layers described in Vedic teachings as koshas (KOH-shuh). Koshas are energetic sheaths that range from dense to increasingly lighter degrees of subtlety. The koshas are not separate objects, but varying qualities of intensity in the spectrum of the whole energy body. Think of the atmosphere around our Earth. Near the surface, the air is dense. Our lungs can operate efficiently here. But as you climb higher, maybe to the peak of a 14,000 mountain in Colorado, the air is much less dense. It is lighter and finer. Breathing is more difficult because we are drawing in much less oxygen than in lower altitudes. Traveling still higher up in the atmosphere, the density of air is increasingly lighter. When we travel by jet airplane at 30,000 feet, we need an oxygenated and pressurized environment to breathe and survive. Just like our atmosphere, our energetic body is also made up of a spectrum of energetic densities.

You can also compare the human energetic body to a spectrum of light or sound frequency. When you look at the colors of the rainbow, the color red vibrates at a much slower rate and lower frequency than the color violet. Similarly, fluctuating vibrations create the sounds we hear. The faster the sound wave travels, the higher the pitch. Slower sound waves produce lower pitched sounds.

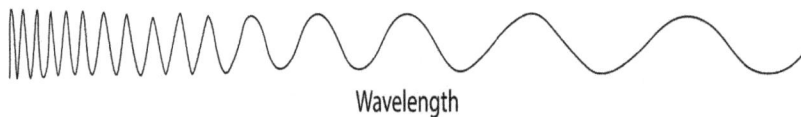

Wavelength

Our human body is comprised of energetic layers of frequencies in much the same way. Our physical body is the densest layer, vibrating at a lower slower frequency. Our breath is comprised of a lighter density. Our thoughts, feelings, emotions, knowledge, intuitions, and spiritual experiences vibrate at successively lighter frequencies.

Try this. Right now, sing the lowest note you can make. Make a low, deep sound. Hear it and feel it vibrate inside your body. Now progressively sing the highest note you can make. Make a light, high sound. Hear it and feel how it vibrates. Now compare the two sounds. They sounded different and they felt much different in your body. The low note is a slower vibration. The high note is a higher vibration. The energetic spectrum of our human subtle body is like that. The physical body has a lower, slower vibration than the breath. The breath vibrates slower than the mind, and so on. Each kosha vibrates at a different rate.

Purify

Pranayama purifies the mind, body, and spirit.

Each kosha or energetic layer provides foundational support for the successive, gradually lighter layers of the energy body. The physical body, annamaya kosha (AH-nah-my-uh), provides a platform and support for the breath body, pranamaya kosha (PRA-nah-my-uh). The breath body supports the mental body, manomaya kosha (mah-NOH-my-uh). The mental body supports the body of high wisdom and intuition, vijnanamaya kosha (vig-NAH-nuh-my-uh). The wisdom body supports the causal or bliss body, anandamaya kosha (AH-nun-duh-my-uh). At the same time, all the layers of the pranic body support one another. They are interdependent.

Unity

Our breath weaves an intimate thread, intertwining among all of our thoughts, feelings, emotions, and experiences. All is connected through the breath.

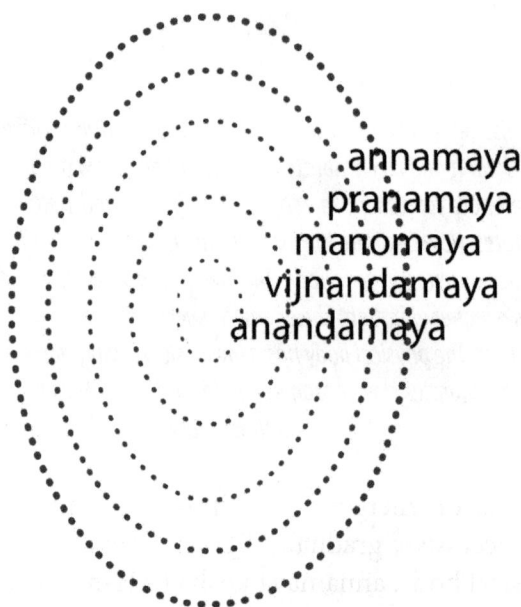

annamaya
pranamaya
manomaya
vijnandamaya
anandamaya

Koshas

Annamaya kosha is the denser, gross layer, and is comprised of our physical body. It is also called the food body, because it is dependent upon food, water, and air.

Pranamaya kosha is the breath body. This layer of our energy body is subtler than the physical body. In our daily life, in yoga practice, and in our pranayama practice, we focus primarily on the body and the breath – the annamaya kosha and the pranamaya kosha. We significantly expand our awareness of the pranamaya kosha, the breath layer, as we explore prana and yogic breathing techniques.

Our physical body, and our pranic, or breath body, provide the foundation and vehicle through which we experience lighter and subtler energies. These increasingly lighter layers of energy;

manomaya kosha, vijnanamaya kosha, and anandamaya kosha, are where we experience awareness of our thoughts, feelings, intuitions, spirituality, and deep blissful states.

· · ·

Developing the ability to discern the qualities of your energetic layers, the koshas, is valuable in pranayama; but most importantly, it can help you develop a better understanding of yourself and others. When you find yourself reacting strongly to a situation in your life as we all do from time to time, try to take a moment to reflect and determine what layer of the body is charged up. For example, dealing with a frustrating performance on the golf course can elicit a physical response. Throwing, breaking, and/or pounding the ground with the golf club shows that annamaya kosha is getting much energy, and perhaps drowning out the subtler layers. But in a different situation, perhaps after a frustrating swing, the same individual may calmly scrutinize the situation, analyze the performance issue, and formulate a plan to achieve a better result in the future. In this case, the mind is doing its job beautifully. Manomaya kosha is receiving an effective amount of energy while the other koshas remain stable and balanced.

When our entire human organism is healthy, our pranic layers work together in a perfectly balanced energetic spectrum. Maintaining harmony and balance is key. The next time you begin to feel the least bit out of balance, pause, be still, and breathe slowly and deeply. Tune in, listen, observe, and take note. Allow the "squeaky wheel to get the grease." Is it your physical body, mind, emotions, high wisdom or spiritual self that is calling out for your attention? What layer needs to be brought into balance? At first you may not decipher the source of your imbalance, but the process of taking time to observe will strengthen your awareness and lead to greater insights. Remember, '*energy flows where awareness goes.*' Be patient. Your rewards will be well worth your efforts. Discipline and progress will evolve steadily over time. You are on the right track.

Pranic Awareness

Understanding the koshas and five vayus gives us an invaluable platform for increasing our awareness of prana. Our human organism is comprised of interdependent, multidimensional energies. Our energetic layers, described as the five koshas, are all permeated by prana. We can use pranic awareness and optimize the flow of pranic energy to access greater knowledge, wisdom, balance, and pleasures in life. For example, we feel and experience prana as intuitive insights in the vijnanamaya kosha. But if the lower, denser layers of the annamaya and manomaya koshas are out of balance or disturbed, we may not be able to discern the more subtle pulsations of prana in the lighter vijnanamaya kosha. The intuitive insight may still happen, but it goes unnoticed because our pranic awareness is diverted or blocked. As we strengthen, balance, and regulate the flow of prana through a healthy physical body and mind; the higher and lighter frequencies of prana in the vijnanamaya and ananandamaya koshas become more accessible to our awareness and available to help us live joyful, balanced, and vibrant lives.

Any of the koshas can become imbalanced. For example, we all have met people that seem to be driven by their mental prowess, the pranas comprising the manomaya kosha. They are brainy, quick-witted, and can probably make a strong case and out-argue just about anyone on any topic. High mental ability serves us well when we can also draw upon our physical, intuitive, and spiritual qualities. There comes a point when a person overly dominant in the manomaya kosha can seem like an annoying know-it-all, and unpleasant to be around. But a person with a very strong pranic field in the manomaya kosha, who is also balanced with a strong physical body, strong abilities to empathize and understand emotional pranas, and high spiritual understanding, is someone you love to be around. They are balanced. They attract people to them. They radiate loving, inspiring energies and share their presence with the rest of us.

Embrace

Wrap yourself up in breath like you are giving yourself a giant hug.

The practice of pranayama helps achieve a balance between the denser, physical body, and the higher layers of the mind, intellect, emotions, and spirit. This is because the pranamaya kosha, the breath layer, lies between body and mind. Breath is the bridge linking the body and mind layers. The practice of pranayama sends vital prana within the vast network of nadis through concentrated hubs of energy at our chakra centers, and on throughout all the physical, mental, intellectual, and spiritual layers of our energetic body. By experiencing the subtle variations of our pranic energies in our physical body via the five vayus we can gain knowledge about the quality of our pranic flow. For example, say the samana vayu (sideways and circular energy in our abdominal region) seems congested, stagnant, or weak. By combining physical means, perhaps by practicing certain yoga asanas, and also practicing conscious breathing techniques; we can take action to dissolve blockages, release stagnation, and increase a healthy flow of samana vayu in the midsection of the body. This in turn promotes healthy pranic flow throughout the entire physical body, and also throughout the lighter, subtler layers of intelligence, wisdom, and bliss. Over time, imbalanced pranic flow can lead to ill health and disease. Balanced pranic flow achieves optimal health, vitality, and a vibrant quality of life.

. . .

I grew up in a time when the saying "seeing is believing" was often the last word. If you could see it, then it must be true. But how many times have you observed a person, place, or thing, but felt that something was not quite right? That something was not entirely congruent? Pay attention. Observe. Discern. Allow access to your higher, intelligent layers of vijnanamaya kosha. Learn to listen to your intuitive insights, or "that little voice inside your head," and your gut reactions.

Bridge

Pranayama is a gateway to meditation.

Try this exercise for expanding your perception and strengthening your discernment. The next time you pick up a magazine, take a close look at the images, and notice how they may have been altered to affect your perception. The photo of the cover model has likely been airbrushed, trimmed down, elongated, and polished. Maybe a photograph has been compiled from several different images, altered to appeal to you in some way—like taking the face of one person and superimposing it onto the body of another? If the magazine is a food, décor, or hobby publication, how has the subject been altered visually to attract you? Would you pick up the magazine if the image had not been altered?

Pranayama can help us keep the higher layers of perception, wisdom, and intuition operating in the foreground of our conscious awareness. Conscious breathing helps us strengthen the currents through the physical body, mind, and higher subtle energetic layers so that our entire spectrum of awareness is available. Pranayama truly leads to expanded perception. You could say it broadens our bandwidth!

What is Pranayama?

A common definition for pranayama (prah-nah-YAH-muh) is "breath control." While controlling the breath is an important component, pranayama encompasses far more than just breathing exercises. Pranayama is comprised from the Sanskrit words, *prana* and *ayama*, which can mean extend, prolong, stretch, restrain, regulate, and expand in time and dimension. Prana is the subtle energy force within the breath. When practicing pranayama, we literally expand all the dimensions of prana, vital life force in all its forms, from gross to subtle, throughout the fullest spectrum of human experience – physical, mental, emotional, and spiritual.

Countless rishis, sages, and scholars have devoted lifetimes toward understanding prana and developing the practices of pranayama. One of our most divine transmitters of sacred knowledge is Rama Jyoti Vernon, a modern-day sage, yogi, and beloved teacher, who beautifully and simply defines pranayama in this way: *"Pra is constant bringing forth. Na is the infinite cosmic vibration. Ya is yeah! Ma is the physical realm of nature of which we are made of, the 3D, the Earth, you. Pranayama is joyfully bringing forth the eternal, infinite cosmos through you!"*

Pranayama is the act of breathing while maintaining keen awareness. By remaining alert and conscious, we can control the breath to intentionally evoke healthy, beneficial changes in ourselves. Pranayama purifies the nadis and energizes the flow of prana, strengthening our physical, mental, emotional, and spiritual vitality. In pranayama practice, we use our awareness, breath, and physical techniques to clear away obstructions in our mental, emotional, and physical bodies so that all aspects of ourselves achieve optimal health and balance. There is a direct connection between our breath and our nervous system. When we learn to harmonize the rhythms of our breath through pranayama, we balance our nerves, our senses, and our mind. We maximize and increase the quantity of our precious prana to experience abundant energy, radiant health, and a highly vibrant quality of life.

Medical research has conclusively proven many benefits of practicing conscious, rhythmic breathing. Pranayama is a viable treatment modality, and a common component in integrative approaches for treating numerous serious diseases. For example, pranayama classes are offered in many cancer treatment centers. Medical research shows that pranayama improves fatigue, sleep disturbance, stress, anxiety, depression, and quality of life in patients undergoing cancer treatment. Forms of pranayama

Balance

Try mirroring inhales with exhales... equal breath in and out. Balance your breath, balance your life.

practices are found in schools, recovery centers, pain clinics, sports performance centers, businesses, and elder care facilities. The applications are endless.

Pranayama is foundational to mindfulness practices and meditation. The first step and essential component in any mindful, meditative process is concentrating and regulating the breath. The simple process of observing the breath, conscious breathing, improves concentration and reduces stress.

One easy breathing practice used in mindfulness meditation is counting breaths. It is a technique that is highly effective in easing into a meditation practice. Try it. Close your eyes, inhale and exhale slowly, and silently count 1. Inhale, exhale, and count 2. Inhale, exhale, and count 3. Count your breaths in this way until you reach 27. Then continue to slowly breathe and count in reverse back down to 1. If you miss a count, start again at 1.

Pranayama calms the nervous system. Stressful conditions activate the sympathetic nervous system, putting you into a tense state of high alert. This state is beneficial when you need to think and react quickly, as you would in responding to an emergency or life-threatening situation. But once the tense situation has passed, you need to remain alert, but lose the tension. Unfortunately, we tend to hold on to stress. Most of us operate with a constant undercurrent of stress as the backstory of our lives. We are continually bombarded with stress-triggering information and circumstances seemingly out of our control. Our sympathetic nervous system stays habitually active and hyper stimulated. This undercurrent of stress is a cause of physical, mental, and emotional dis-ease.

Pranayama helps us achieve balance by slowing down the rhythm of our nerves activating the relaxation response mechanisms of the parasympathetic nervous system. By learning to consciously control your breath, you begin to master your thoughts, feelings, and reactions to life's situations. Pranayama helps you move between action and relaxation, while maintaining control and awareness at all times. We can consciously activate more energy and alertness by practicing a rapid and strong breathing technique, and we can also slow down the breath to lower our heart rate and relax.

Regular practice of pranayama allows you to develop a broad range of breath rhythms, which allows you to operate effectively and remain in control throughout the ebbs and flows of events and circumstances in life. Sometimes we need to react quickly, keep our presence of mind, and be effective in highly charged situations. Other times we need to slow down, appreciate and absorb the abundant beauty, joy, and love all around us. Pranayama gives us the ability to navigate our lives vibrantly across a very broad bandwidth with grace and ease.

Pranayama can energize you, revitalize you, purify you, heal you, and help you overcome obstacles in life. During times of stress, anxiety, and fear, pranayama can help you calm and stabilize. In times of peace and harmony, pranayama can help you find even greater dimensions of tranquility and bliss. With consistent pranayama practice your prana will flow smoothly throughout all layers of your being. Vibrant health, happiness, serenity, rejuvenation, radiance, and immense love are the rewards.

. . .

My grandmother was not a yogi, but she ,as with most other grandmothers, told her beloved ones to ". . . take a deep breath and count to ten," before speaking or acting out in anger. This simple little piece of folk wisdom contains some pretty amazing advice for managing thoughts, emotions, and actions by controlling the breath.

Prana: Vital Life Force Energy

Connect

Connect your thoughts, emotions, body, spirit and soul through your breath.

Pranayama and Yoga

Over two thousand years ago, a revered Vedic sage called Patanjali compiled an epic work called The Yoga Sutras of Patanjali, which forms the basis of yoga as we know it today. In the Yoga Sutras, Patanjali lays out the eight limbs of yoga, or the eightfold path. These eight steps act as a roadmap for living a conscious, meaningful, and highly vibrant life. The eight steps are meant to build upon one another and form a progression: Yama, Niyama, Asana, Pranayama, Pratyahara, Dharana, Dhyana, and Samadhi.

Yama literally means "restraint". Yamas are ethical rules, similar to the Ten Commandments. They are ahimsa, nonviolence; satya, truthfulness; asteya, non-stealing; bramrya, control and moderation of the senses; and aparigraha, non-possessiveness.

Niyama means rules, laws or observances. The niyamas are saucha, purity; santosha, contentment; tapas, self-discipline and dedication; svadhyaya, self-study; and ishvara pranidhana, surrender of personal will and celebration of the spiritual.

Asanas are the physical poses. Most of us in the Western world view yoga as the physical practice, but asana is only one of the eight limbs of yoga.

Pranayama is controlling and expanding life force energy through the breath.

Pratyahara is quieting the senses and drawing them in from the outer world.

Dharana is concentration. Dharana is the ability to focus the mind's attention on one point or task without becoming distracted.

Dhyana is meditation. Dhyana is a meditative state with longer, deeper, sustained concentration without distraction.

Samadhi is union with the Divine. It is self-realization, superconsciousness, celebration of the spiritual, and is the ultimate goal of yoga.

Each limb of yoga describes qualities and attributes that stand alone. Anyone would benefit by observing just one of the eight limbs; but we can clearly see that Patanjali laid out a path which progressively unfolds and leads to higher aspects of the self, and ultimately, to spiritual enlightenment. He starts out by giving some guidelines for how to be a good, clean, and moral person with social skills to benefit self and society. From there, how to achieve a strong, flexible body. It's interesting to take a look at just where pranayama fits within the progression along the eightfold path. Pranayama is sandwiched in-between physical asana and the subtle and refined practices of pratyahara, dharana, dhyana, and samadhi. Learning to control and expand the quantum of prana within the body leads to inner sensory awareness, concentration, meditation, and self-realization.

Basic Mechanics
of Breathing

*I*n the simplest physical terms, our breathing brings in a steady supply of oxygen and eliminates carbon dioxide. Through our respiratory system, we receive oxygen from the air into our lungs, bloodstream, and cells. Carbon dioxide is released from the cells, returned to the bloodstream, and carried to the lungs before being expelled into the air.

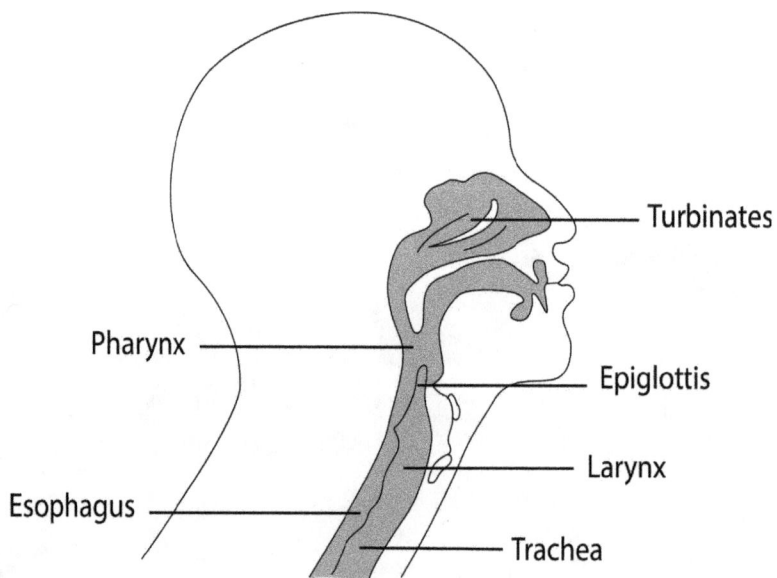

Nasal Flow

Our nostrils provide a passageway for air to enter the body. Nostrils are lined with hairs that filter and warm the air as it flows in, trapping dust and debris. Air enters deeper into the nasal mucous membranes, where it is further moistened and cleansed by cilia, microscopic hairs. The air then enters the nasal cavities, where it is swirled around, warmed, and further humidified. The prepared air then travels down through the pharynx, larynx, and trachea, where it is further cleansed by more tiny cilia.

The air then travels down and branches into either bronchus as it enters the lobes of the lungs. The air is routed through increasingly numerous and gradually smaller conduits of the tree-like bronchi network. The air finally reaches the end of the bronchioles and enters the alveoli, tiny air sacs. In the alveoli, oxygen travels through alveolar-capillary membranes to enter the blood. Carbon dioxide transfers from the blood, into the air sacs, and travels back out of the lungs through the bronchioles, bronchi, trachea, nasal passages, and finally the nostrils.

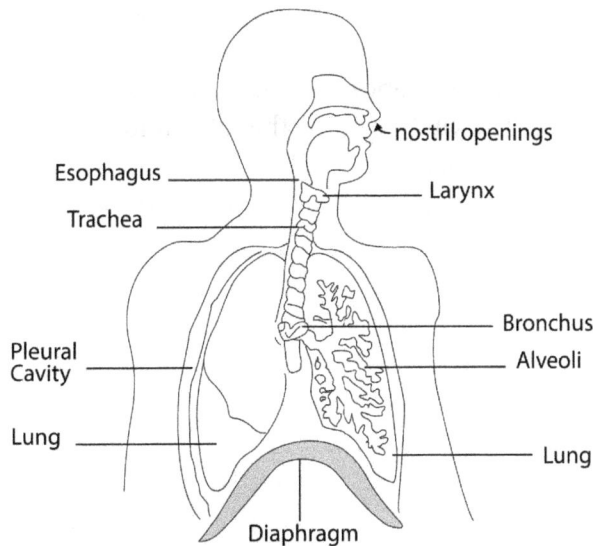

Respiratory System

Basic Mechanics of Breathing

The lungs are housed in the thoracic cavity, protected by the ribcage, and supported underneath by the respiratory diaphragm. The diaphragm does most of the movement of breathing. It is a large, dome-shaped muscle sheath that separates the thoracic cavity from the abdominal cavity. During inspiration the diaphragm contracts, flattens out, and draws downward. This action widens the ribcage, increases volume, and lowers pressure in the thoracic cavity to allow air to rush in. During normal exhalation, the diaphragm relaxes and returns to its original domed shape, allowing the air to flow out as the lungs deflate, similar to the way an inflated balloon deflates when released.

Volume and Rate

The average healthy adult breathes in half a liter of air with each normal inhale. This is the tidal volume. There is also a reserve capacity, which is the amount of air a person can intentionally breathe in, and also breathe out beyond the tidal volume. The inhalation reserve is about 3 liters, and exhalation reserve is about 1 liter. The vital capacity, the total amount of air the lungs can inhale and exhale, is up to 5.5 liters. Around 1.2 liters of air, the residual volume, always remains in the lungs even after we exhale completely.

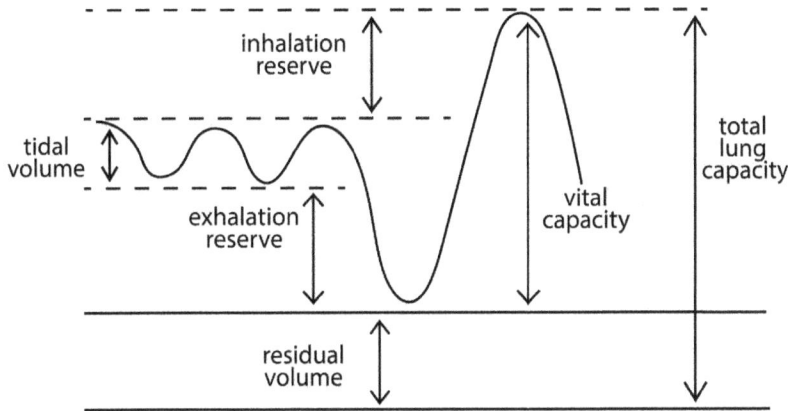

Lung Volumes

Most adults breathe between 12 and 16 breaths per minute. This rate varies significantly, and is influenced by environmental, physical, and emotional conditions and circumstances. During vigorous exercise, the breath rate may climb up to 20-30 breaths per minute, yet during deep meditation the breath rate may slow down to 3 or fewer breaths per minute.

You Have Control

Breathing is regulated by the autonomic nervous system, which also regulates involuntary functions of the body such as heart rate, body temperature, and blood pressure. If we paid no attention whatsoever to our breath, we would continue to breathe automatically, thanks to the autonomic nervous system.

Of all the involuntary systems governed by the autonomic nervous system, we have the ability to consciously control only one, the breath. We can change our breath rate and volume at will. By controlling our breath we can change our heartbeat, blood pressure, and other bodily functions ruled by the autonomic nervous system. The breath carries prana. We can consciously use our breath to affect our body, mind, emotions, and subtle energies by influencing the flow of prana.

The autonomic nervous system is made up of the sympathetic and parasympathetic nervous systems. The sympathetic nervous system is associated with stimulation. It prepares the body and mind for action. The parasympathetic nervous system is associated with a relaxed state. The body and mind are influenced by the nervous system that is dominant at any given time. When the sympathetic system is heightened, the body is ready to spring into action at any moment, in a state of high tension or acute stress. This is called the "fight or flight" effect. The nerves are highly stimulated and ready to respond to a perceived threatening situation. When the parasympathetic system is active, the body can rest and rejuvenate. The body is not preparing to react to danger or assault, but is stable and calm. When the sympathetic and parasympathetic nervous systems become unbalanced, prana flow is disturbed. Prana can become erratic, excessive, and unstable; or diminished, blocked, and stuck resulting in ill health. Stress overloads our nervous system, causes imbalance, and keeps the sympathetic nervous system continually active and operating on high alert. When the autonomic nervous system is balanced, our vital bodily systems function within a healthy, nurtured environment, and the body can operate smoothly and efficiently.

We activate the parasympathetic nervous system primarily by stimulating the vagus nerve. Many pranayama techniques are specifically designed to stimulate the vagus nerve, producing a parasympathetic response. The vagus nerve acts as a reset mechanism after a stressful event. It sends impulses to the brain, signaling there is no threat present. The sympathetic nervous system can let go and allow the parasympathetic nervous system to come online. Controlling the breath, especially slowing the rate and increasing the breath volume, stimulates the vagus nerve and activates the parasympathetic system. One of the easiest ways to stimulate the vagus nerve is diaphragmatic breathing. Simply taking long, deep breaths from the belly strengthens the vagal tone and activates the parasympathetic nervous system. Heart rate and blood pressure lowers, stress response subsides, and the body and mind can function calmly, naturally, and vibrantly. Prana flows steadily and smoothly, and you experience vibrant physical, mental, emotional, and spiritual vitality.

Consistent

Practice pranayama regularly and rhythmically.

. . .

Sometimes life can feel overwhelming. Much is completely out of your control, but you always have the ability to control your breath. No matter what the circumstance, conscious control of your breathing will help balance your body, mind, and emotions. Practice mindfully controlling your breath in everything you do: driving, cooking, writing, singing, running, thinking —you get the picture!

Basic Mechanics of Breathing

*Nurture
continuous
awareness of
your breath as
you go about
your daily
activities. Simply
observe and feel
the breath flow
in and out all
day long.*

Breathe Through the Nose or Mouth?

Most pranayama practices focus on breathing through the nostrils, and unless specifically noted, assume nostril breathing. In addition to the cleansing, warming, and humidifying processes in the nasal region, there are important energetic, pranic reasons for breathing through the nostrils. The nostrils are important elements of the main ida and pingala nadi channels. Andre van Lysebeth refers to nostrils as "pure pranic antennae." Prana enters and exits the body through the cone-shaped antennae, the passageways of ida and pingala nadis. The potent mixture of air and prana stimulates the ajna chakra center, just behind the eyebrow point, associated with the pineal gland in the brain. The higher energy centers in the body are activated as breath enters and exits through the nasal passages. As you practice conscious awareness while breathing through the nostrils, you will begin to feel prana rise up from the denser centers in the base of the spine, through gradually lighter centers up into the eyebrow center. Sensations of lightness, expansiveness, and clarity accompany mindful nostril breathing as the upper centers of the pranic body are stimulated.

Try breathing through the mouth for several minutes. Just observe. Do not try to evoke any particular sensation or feeling. Simply breathe through your mouth and notice how you feel. Now close your lips and breathe slowly through the nostrils for several minutes.

Again, simply observe the sensations and feelings of breathing deeply through the nostrils. Now return to normal, spontaneous breathing and notice the differences in the sensations you experienced with nostril breathing versus mouth breathing.

It is also important to try to be aware of the nostril openings while practicing pranayama. As you develop and refine your pranic awareness, you will experience more sensitivity in the nostrils. You will learn to consciously control the flaring of the nostrils as your pranayama practice evolves.

Try it now. Flare your nostril openings and soften them a few times. It may seem silly at first, but try it a few times. Flare them open then soften them a bit. Now try to control the flaring action. Make the flare slow and steady. Try to refine the very subtle movement involved in flaring the nostril rims. Play with it. Try flaring just the very tips, then try flaring just the mid-section of the nostril, followed by the upper parts.

Try stiffening and strengthening the inner walls of the nostrils as you breathe in and out. Feel more prana concentrate inside the nostrils and absorb into the body. Try dilating the nostrils when you breathe in. Relax them as you breathe out.

Remember to pay attention to your nostrils in all of the pranayama techniques. You will increase the amount of oxygen coming into your body and also absorb more prana into your subtle energy layers.

Basic Mechanics of Breathing

Fundamentals:
Let's Get Started

*B*reathe in, breathe out, repeat. What could be more straight-forward and simple? By now, we recognize that this natural act of breathing, practiced with conscious awareness can open portals into higher layers of our human energetic anatomy. Ancient yogis, rishis and seers spent lifetimes mastering access into these realms and the practice of pranayama was a fundamental platform for their exploration of finer, subtle, sublime frequencies. In our daily lives, we may not ever reach the heightened awareness of those vedic sages, but we can utilize their basic pranayama techniques to enhance our health, happiness and well being.

Set the Stage

Many pranayamas can be practiced anytime, anywhere, while others will require you to find a clean, quiet, and private area. The most important consideration, no matter where you will be practicing, is to first create an internal space, a conscious intention for your pranayama practice. Perhaps setting the internal space simply means that you choose to be fully present and vitally aware of focusing on your breathing technique. Our minds are accustomed to overwhelming amounts of external stimuli, and it may present a challenge to block out distractions and stay focused on your pranayama for any length of time. With practice, your attention span will increase, but the first step is to set a clear intention that you will devote a certain amount of time, or number of rounds, to your pranayama exercise. Set a reasonable goal, perhaps just for a few minutes, and then muster up the discipline to follow through on your promise to yourself to focus on your pranayama technique. Remember that *energy flows where awareness goes*. If you focus your awareness on your breathing practice, your pranic energies will become stronger and your concentration will improve. Before too long, you will extend the duration and quality of your sessions with comfort and ease.

Quiet

Pranayama quiets the mind.

Physical Place

Ideally, the space you choose for your pranayama practice should have plenty of clean, fresh air. Try not to practice in dusty, smoky areas, or where there are volatile fumes or strong odors. It is best to be protected from loud noises, excess motion, and external distractions. An important consideration is that you will be balancing your internal pranas, so strong external energies can work against your practice if you have to work too hard to "tune out" environmental chaos. Try to find a clean, quiet space. However, with practice, you will develop the ability to find quiet internal space pretty much anywhere, anytime. For example, there are many pranayamas you can practice while standing in line at the supermarket, sitting and waiting for an appointment, and even while driving.

I like to lightly spritz some essential oil into the air just before I practice. Uplifting scents such as geranium, citrus, or mint are nice for energizing practices; and soothing scents such as lavender, rose, sandalwood, or neroli are nice for calming practices. You may want to experiment with different aromas for your practice. Just make sure you keep the scent very, very light—just the faintest hint of essence. Simply place a few drops of essential oil into a clean spray bottle of water, and lightly spritz.

. . .

One of my favorite objects is my aromatherapy diffuser. Basically, it is a small, ultrasonic humidifier that disperses water vapor into the air. Add a few drops of essential oil to the water and the aroma mist fills the room. Many specialty sites online carry them, but in a pinch, you can use an ordinary cool mist humidifier from the drugstore.

Squeaky Clean

Your physical environment should be as clean and uncluttered as possible. For example, if you will plan to practice at your messy office desk cluttered with papers and files, take a moment to organize and stack them neatly, and perhaps place them to the side before you begin. The act of organizing and cleaning sets in motion a quality of purity and mindful awareness that will help balance your internal pranas. Before long, if you are consistent with your pranayama practice, your nadi channels will become strengthened and purified, and you will find yourself naturally maintaining a clean, pure work and home environment. You will want your external environment to support your internal environment.

Keep your clothes and body clean. As your grandmother may have said, "cleanliness is next to godliness." Pranayama helps you access higher life force energies, physically, mentally, emotionally, and spiritually. Dirt, dust, and debris are energy traps. Pranayama practice is like cleaning the film from a smudged window, changing the air filter, or doing a deep spring cleaning. Starting with a clean and neat body will make it easier to cleanse and purify your subtle energy layers.

It is a good practice to regularly cleanse the nostrils by using a neti pot. You can find neti pots in most drug stores and super-markets. The nasal passages are cleansed by gently pouring a mild, warm saline solution through one nostril, allowing the stream of saline to flow out of the other nostril.

Try also to eat "clean" foods. Avoid heavy, greasy food and pro-cessed foods. Eat foods high in prana such as nutritious fresh fruits, vegetables, and whole grains. If you eat animal products, try to avoid red meat, and instead, gravitate toward fresh fish and organic poultry. Try to steer away from foods that may produce excess mucous and phlegm, such as heavy dairy products.

Practice on an empty stomach. Try to eat two hours before your pranayama practice, or wait until after. Some techniques require an empty tummy due to physical and energetic activation of the navel and abdominal regions. If the body is focused on digesting food, it cannot fully support the pranayama technique. If you practice pranayama while the body is trying to digest, neither the pranayama nor digestion will be optimal, and may even be harmful.

When is the Best Time to Practice?

If you wait for the perfect time, it may never come. So jump in right away and commit to practicing daily. Ideally choose the same time each day and stick to it. It is good to give yourself a goal of 40 days of daily practice. Find the calendar or calendar

Prepare

Clear some space, establish yourself in stillness and be ready for amazing awakenings.

app that you like to use, and set up a reminder for yourself. If you skip a day, then start again until you practice consistently for 40 days. Daily, consistent practice is the goal. Just start, your rewards will be vast!

Early morning is a traditional time to practice pranayama, ideally just before the sun rises. At this time of the day the natural pranas of the earth are awakening, rising up, and gaining strength and vitality for the day. Animals begin to awaken, birds sing, the sun's rays begin to bathe and illuminate the earth, and our own prana naturally begins to rise from sleep. Your mind and body are fresh, rested, and without distraction. Set your alarm a bit earlier than usual, and try an early morning practice for 40 days. Before long, you may not need an external alarm clock. Your body will naturally wake up from sleep early in the morning, looking forward to an infusion of beautiful prana to begin the day in perfect harmony with the natural pranic rhythms of the earth.

Similarly, the time around sunset is an ideal time to practice, as pranic energies shift from activity to restfulness. Balancing, soothing pranayamas are ideal at dusk, to ease the transition from the activities of the day and to prepare your body and mind for a pleasant and restful sleep.

But really, any time can be the best time for you to practice. It's important to practice consistently, even for a few minutes. Apply yourself. There are infinite possibilities to find a few minutes to devote to your breathing practice throughout the day. As you develop a steady, consistent pranayama practice you will soon find that your awareness of breath becomes second nature. As you are aware of your breath more of the time, you will feel calm, centered, balanced, and focused. Your mental and physical strength and vitality will improve as your pranic energies balance and flow rhythmically and steadily. Practice every day, several times a day.

. . .

I practice pranayama and meditation every morning, but it was not always easy to discipline myself to practice consistently upon arising. The bit of advice that worked for me came from Erich Schiffmann. He said, "...give yourself permission to sit up comfortably in bed, in your pajamas, warm and comfy with the covers over your legs, and begin." In his unique personal style, he said, "Just start practicing. Make it eeeaaaaaaasy." Erich's approach made finding a time to practice easy and consistent, and helped me establish a routine. Now pranayama and meditation are essential to my daily routine and I look forward to practicing every day. Thanks, Erich!

Posture

The physical body is the supporting structure, platform, and foundation for pranayama. Your breath needs the support and alignment of your body. Over time, most of us developed habits that affect the integrity of our posture. But, the positive news is that, as you become more aware of how you are breathing, and begin to breathe consciously and steadily, your posture will naturally begin to align to more effectively support you. We have learned that the body is made up of energetic layers, all supporting one another. The physical body, annamaya kosha, supports the breath body, pranamaya kosha, and at the same time the breath supports the physical body. It works both ways. With

Attitude

Pranic vibrations produce thoughts in the mind. Nurture good prana. Insist on good prana. Accept only the highest pranas. Live with awesome attitude.

consistent pranayama practice, your posture will develop structural integrity because you need to have physical strength and alignment for optimal breathing. You will cultivate greater body awareness and vitality as your circulation, respiration, and overall strength naturally improve. With proper alignment and good posture, you will find yourself feeling and looking stronger, happier, healthier, and more radiant.

. . .

Try this simple experiment. Slump your body, let your belly go flaccid and let your head hang heavy. Try breathing deeply while your body is in this shape. It's kind of difficult to take a big breath, isn't it? Now sit up straight and tall, but keep your shoulders and neck relaxed. Sit with good posture and breathe deeply. It feels better now, doesn't it? Simple, deep breathing with a straight spine and good postural alignment will help you build strength and stamina.

Establish a Firm Base

Whether sitting, standing, or reclining, feel a secure connection to the surface below you. Every part of you touching the surface beneath is part of your root – your base. If you are sitting, feel your hips and thighs press down, and be aware of the sensation of connection with the firm support below you. If you are sitting in a chair, feel your feet press into the floor and be aware of the surface of your back against the back of the chair. Develop a sense of feeling securely established, grounded, and stable.

See
*Master your
breath and see
the divine in
everything.*

Developing a strong sense of being rooted, grounded, and stable may take a little time and practice for some of us. If we are overly active in our mental and emotional layers, experiencing a particularly stressful day, or feeling especially distracted or consumed by an issue in life, it's important to send some extra awareness to the process of grounding and stabilizing. A good way to begin is to quiet down and breathe slowly, feeling into the apana vayu, downward moving prana from the navel to the perineum. Simply by being aware of apana vayu, you begin to stabilize and bring more balance to all the pranas in your body.

Keep a Straight but Relaxed Spine

Begin by lengthening and straightening your spine. Even if you are practicing while lying down, encourage your backbone to slightly elongate. Notice what happens when you straighten your spine. Some of us will adopt a sort of military rigidity, like standing at full attention. If you slip into a habit of tensing up or becoming rigid, take a moment to loosen up, shake your shoulders, and move your head from side to side. Come back again. Focus awareness and intention on staying fully relaxed while allowing the spine to naturally grow taller.

Now relax your shoulders, slightly lift your sternum, and draw your skull back just a little. This may sound tricky, but it can be effortless and natural when you send your awareness to your upper body. Many of us have a holding pattern of rounding the shoulders and caving in the chest. Gently lift the sternum as you roll the shoulders back and down, so the front of your chest

*Breathe deeply
into the depths
of your soul. Feel
the luminous
glow of divine
life force
illuminate the
central channel
of your spine.
Radiate your
beautiful love
into infinity.*

naturally broadens and expands. Keep a neutral, level chin and lightly draw the skull back a little, and feel the back of your neck elongate. Relax and breathe easy.

Discover Three Stretch Zones in Your Spine

Most of us have tight backs, and it can be challenging to feel just what area of the back is holding tension, keeping you stiff, stuck and misaligned. It may be helpful to focus awareness into three distinct areas in the back. Let's begin to explore.

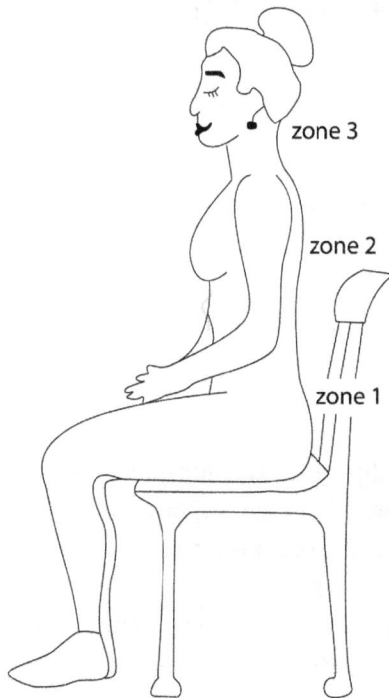

Three Stretch Zones

Begin by sitting comfortably in a chair, or on a cushion on the floor. The first stretch zone spans between the hips to the lower ribs, your lumbar spine. Elongate this region by first anchoring your hips down into the surface below you to form a secure base. As you breathe slowly in and out, feel your lower ribs elevate up and away from the hips. Keep secure and stable in the base, then breathe fully to elongate the midsection. Try to keep this region lengthened. Keep lengthening from the hips to the lower ribs, while keeping the chest, shoulders, neck, and head relaxed. It may help to first get in touch with the grounding sensations of apana vayu, downward moving energy from the navel to the perineum. Become aware of samana vayu, the inward and circular energetic movement in the midsection. As you exhale, feel your midsection draw in around the navel as the sides of your waist elongate, your hips press down, and your lower ribs lift up.

The next zone is from the lower ribs to the base of the neck, your thoracic spine. Many of us hold a good deal of tension here, and it can be difficult to feel expansive and open in this area. Imagine this section becoming very flexible, very "bendy". With your lower back elongated, expand through the collarbones, lower your shoulder blades, and very softly encourage your shoulder blades to draw toward one another behind you. Breathe softly and try to relax your shoulders a little more. Now, keep the lower back and midsection elongated, head lifted, and separate your shoulder blades. Stretch them apart from one another on your back. Do this several times, pulling the shoulder blades together, then expanding them apart. Be still for a moment, then breathe fully while expanding, and relax the entire region between the neck and the lower ribs. Do this several minutes, and remember to also keep the lower back elongated. This stretch zone is the dwelling place of prana vayu. Prana vayu is the force that brings air into the body and it feels expansive. As you inhale, feel the front chest, side chest, and back chest expand. As you exhale, keep the seat grounded, midsection elongated, and feel the chest area relax and slightly deflate.

The third stretch zone is from the base of the neck to the back of the skull, your cervical spine. Keeping your lower back elongated, your mid back open, and your shoulders relaxed, begin to lift your sternum as you draw your chin back slightly. You should keep the chin relatively level and, perhaps ever so slightly low-

Lift

*Lift your pranas
very high up
through your
spine with your
beautiful breath.*

Pleasure

Breathe in only joy, light, and happiness. Astound yourself with the pleasures of breath.

ered, as you draw the chin back. You will feel a slight lengthening from the base of the neck to the back of the skull. The key is keeping the back and torso elongated, yet relaxed, while feeling the cervical spine stretch a bit. Most of us hold a good deal of tension in the back, base of the neck, and upper shoulders. Try to relax and perhaps do a few slow, easy neck rolls, making sure you keep the lower back and midsection active and lifted before resuming your exploration of the cervical spine stretch zone. This area is where we feel udana vayu, upward moving prana. As you inhale, feel vibrant energy rise up through the neck, face, skull, and crown of your head. As you exhale, feel the relaxing, and slightly euphoric sensations, stimulating your senses in the head.

Play with your awareness of these three zones. Notice how each zone feels, moves, stretches, and opens a bit differently from the other areas.

Most of All, Be Comfortable

Your posture should be easy, relaxed, aligned, and comfortable. Remember, your breath influences your physical body and your physical body influences your breath. As you practice pranayama your posture will naturally evolve. Each time you practice, you will become more aware of subtle structural alignments and refinements over time. Be as relaxed and comfortable as you can be each time you practice. Try not to judge yourself. Simply accept where you are and practice with a fresh attitude each and every time. You will be amazed at the positive changes that seem to occur naturally, organically, and effortlessly.

Easy

When you steady
your breath
you steady your
mind.

Easy Does It

Easy, easy, easy. You may be accustomed to working hard to achieve positive outcomes in work, sports, hobbies, and even relationships; but in pranayama practice, working hard is the wrong approach, and can be harmful. In pranayama practice, working gently, slowly and consistently yields positive results. Never, ever strain. Never. Never, ever retain the breath past your comfort zone. Never, ever, period. The linings of your nostrils and lungs are delicate. Pranic flow is delicate. Balancing and purifying your energetic pathways is delicate business. You will progress with steady, consistent, gentle practice. Slow mastery of very simple techniques is the goal. Learn to master a slow, steady, even flow of breath. Master fluid, liquid-like transitions between inhales, exhales, and holds. Master fluidity. Eliminate choppiness and inconsistent breath flow. It is best to practice one or two techniques for weeks or months to develop a depth of awareness of very subtle fluctuations in your energetic field. Some practices will yield immediate sensations of exhilaration or deep bliss. While these sensations are very real and beneficial, it is important to practice a technique consistently over time to begin to unfold the layers of subtle awareness, and to expand your abilities to perceive the very refined and sublime qualities of your higher energies. This takes gentle, steady practice, and time.

Developing Heightened Awareness of Breath

*T*he first step in any conscious breathing, stress reduction, or meditation practice is to simply be aware of your breath. It sounds easy and effortless, and it can be just that straightforward; but if you are unaccustomed to remaining still and tuning out all external distractions and stimulation to direct your attention inward, then you are among the millions of people who will need some time and practice to re-learn this vital life skill.

Breath Awareness

Developing awareness of the breath may seem very easy and natural for some people, but is not so simple for others. Breath awareness requires us to detach a bit and play the role of observer, simultaneously observing and experiencing. Yogis developed extremely refined mental concentration. Their process is based upon mindfully focusing awareness on the breath.

Our breath is an indicator of the state of our nervous system. External events, and those experiences occurring within the mind, influence the patterns, rhythms, and character of our breathing. For example, when something disturbing or upsetting happens, we may gasp, sharply inhale, restrict, or hold the breath.

When we experience profound beauty, love, or pleasure, we may let out a sigh, relax with a long exhale, and breathe smoothly, deeply and evenly.

You can easily experience this for yourself. Sit quietly for a moment and prepare to use your imagination. Imagine that something tragic, shocking, upsetting, or alarming is happening. Observe your breathing pattern, your emotions, and your physical reactions. Did you tense up? Hold your breath? Tighten the chest and throat? Harden your belly?

Next, imagine yourself experiencing something profoundly beautiful, tender, and lovely. Maybe you imagine holding a little baby, smelling a beautiful fragrant flower, watching a magnificent sunset over the ocean, or caressing your true love. Observe your breathing pattern, your emotions, and your physical reactions. Notice the difference in ways you reacted in each experience.

When something in our life, real or imagined, is stressful or unpleasant, we react by constricting our diaphragm and restricting our breath. When we experience pleasure, we soften our diaphragm, relax and slow our breathing.

This breath/emotion relationship works both ways. The breath influences emotions and emotions influence the breath. If constricted, shallow breathing is habitual, then over time a pattern of repeated negative feelings and emotions may develop. If full, deep and even breathing is the predominant pattern, then positive emotional states are supported. As you develop more awareness of your breath, you become more aware of your emotions, thoughts, and feelings. You develop awareness of the interrelationship between breathing and state of mind, and this awareness will lead you toward greater balance in your life.

Cultivate

Cultivate an intimate and profound relationship with your breath and vibrate your love affair deep into the world.

Renew

With each and every breath cycle, fully empty every ounce of breath from your lungs. Relax, soften to receive a flowing wave of a brand new breath, a sparkling infusion of fresh life force energy, and awaken into a brand new beginning.

Essential Breath Awareness Techniques

The following few practices are designed to connect your awareness to the natural rhythms of your breath. Breathing awareness is a foundational process with vast and profound benefits. Heart rate slows, blood pressure lowers, mind becomes calm, concentration improves, parasympathetic nervous system comes online, and prana begins to flow smoothly.

Explore some of the following practices and discover your breath. Even if you are a seasoned meditator, yogi and pranayama practitioner, breath awareness is a continually evolving and deeply dynamic personal process. Developing greater breath awareness is a boundless and eternal evolution, sure to illuminate unlimited possibilities and insights!

Mindful Breath Awareness

In this practice, you will simply observe your natural breath without trying to control or manipulate your breathing in any way. You will find that, by simply directing awareness to your breath, your breathing begins to become steady, slow, natural, and relaxed.

Let's begin. Sit up nice and tall, and place your feet soundly on the floor. You may also practice while comfortably lying down. Relax your face and shoulders. You will breathe in and out of your nostrils, not the mouth. Lightly close your lips, but keep your teeth slightly apart. If you like, you may rest the tip of your tongue lightly behind the upper front teeth. Relax your neck and jaw. Be comfortable.

Explore

Explore the vast and infinite dimensions of breath.

Direct your awareness to your nostrils. Feel your breath flowing into and out of your nostrils. Feel your breath travel in through the nostril openings, travel up the nasal passages, and travel deep into the body. Feel your breath flow out from deep within the body to the top of the nasal passages. Feel your breath flow downward through the nostrils, and feel the breath flow out of the nostril openings into the air in front of your body. Breathe for several minutes, observing the journey of your breath flowing into the body through the nostrils, then gently out again.

Silently describe how the breath feels as it enters the openings of the nostrils, and how it feels as it flows out of the nostril openings. Does the temperature of the breath change? Are there changes in the rate in which it flows? What about the volume of air coming in and out? Do you feel changes in temperature of your breath as it comes in and when it flows out? Is your breath flowing smoothly? Does it feel silky? Or do you feel hesitation, choppiness, roughness, or constriction?

Now be aware of the inner space of your mouth. As your breath flows into and out of your body, what sensations occur inside your mouth? Do the inner cheeks soften and feel hollow? Do you feel expansion between your teeth and the smooth skin lining the mouth? Does your jaw relax or does it hold tension?

Continue to observe and feel the path of your breath and closely feel into your throat area. Experience your throat relax, soften and expand as it receives the breath. Feel a calm release as your breath glides back out again. Observe the upper opening of your throat. Is the breath flowing gently and smoothly through the

Observe

Learn to be a keen observer of your breathing.

throat opening? Do you feel friction there? Relax and feel the breath flow through entire length of your windpipe. Does the breath glide and slide along this passageway? Do you feel dryness or constriction?

Become more aware as your breath flows down and broadens into the chest. Feel your breath expand and softly open into the fullness of the chest. Feel your chest delicately deflate ever so slightly as your breath leaves. Observe your breath gently rise up and flow out of your chest, into the throat, and out of the nostrils.

Next, feel your breath flow deeper down into the lungs. Feel your lungs inflate and expand as the breath comes in. Feel your lungs relax and deflate a little as your breath flows out. Can you feel the lower lobes of your lungs tenderly swell as your breath fills in? Do you feel the lower tips of your lungs relax as your breath flows out?

Feel the breath fill out the rib cage. As the breath ebbs and flows, experience the ribs widen out, then relax in. Feel the lower ribs open and expand as you inhale, and soften as you breathe out. Feel into the lower back ribs and mid back ribs. Can you feel them move, even subtly? Do you feel the rib cage enlarge, then diminish? How do your front ribs and sternum move as you breathe in and out?

Become aware of your breath coming into the abdominal area. As you inhale, keep the ribs quiet and begin to feel the abdomen let go and expand. Do you feel tight or hardened in the belly, or does it feel soft and full? Can you feel your belly relax and deflate as your breath flows out of your body? Do you feel your belly billow and inflate like a balloon as the breath comes in?

Now view the entire journey of your breath as it freely and smoothly pours in from the tips of the nostrils all the way down deep into the belly. Feel the breath linger a bit in the lower belly. Observe as your breath flows up from the belly and floats gently out of the nostrils.

Continue to observe your breathing. Watch and feel your breath smoothly flow from the openings of the nostrils, slowly and evenly traveling downward to linger in the base of the lower belly, then feel your breath gently and naturally return upward and softly leave your body through the openings of your nostrils.

When you are ready to end the practice, take a couple of deep, energizing breaths. Move your fingers and toes, rotate your ankles and wrists, open and close your fists, and scrunch the toes before spreading them wide. Reach your arms over your head and stretch the arms and legs away from one another. Be fully alert and aware of your surroundings. Feel vibrantly present in your physical body. Pause, rest, and notice how you feel.

Expansive Breathing Awareness

This simple breath awareness practice is profoundly soothing, calming, and excellent for reducing anxiety. This breath helps you feel light and open, and helps you cope with challenges in life.

To begin, lie on your back and become comfortable. Close your eyes and allow your body to relax and rest. Try to feel the weight of your body and spine become heavier. Feel the spine being supported by the surface underneath you. It may help to bend your knees and gently press down with the soles of your feet to feel

Joy

Breathe deeply. Don't worry. Be light. Be happy. Take comfort in knowing that all of us, everywhere around our Earth are breathing the same breath. All of us, together. Breathe joyfully. It's what we're all here to do!

the length of your spine. You may keep your knees bent if this helps you feel the surface of your sacrum press into the surface beneath you. Feel secure, stable, and grounded. Relax your arms and allow them to rest comfortably alongside your body.

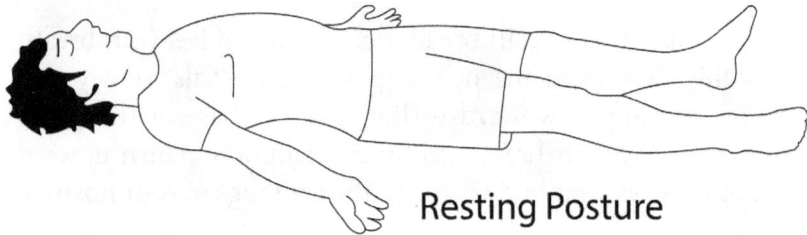

Resting Posture

Slowly breathe in and out of your nostrils. Lips stay together and teeth slightly apart. Notice the nostril openings, and become aware of the breath flowing in and out. Relax and feel the breath drift in and travel deep into the body. Feel your breath flow out of the body through the nostrils.

Soften and relax your belly. Feel your belly expand and become pliable and elastic as the breath flows in. Be aware of your entire abdomen, the front, sides, and back areas. Feel the entire surface of your belly inflate in all directions as you breathe in. Feel your belly deflate just a little as the breath flows out.

Feel into your chest and ribs. Relax. Smooth out the transition between inhaling and exhaling. Soften any choppiness, catching or abruptness. Make your breath form a smooth, deep, even, continuously flowing stream. Feel your chest area inflate larger and larger as the breath comes in. Deflate a little more as the breath flows out.

Feel the entire torso billow, expanding larger and larger in every direction, as more oxygen flows into your body. Feel your body inflate and feel lighter. Keep the feeling of spaciousness and expansiveness as you experience your breath release.

Feel the sensations of expansive breathing without judging or evaluating. There is no right way or wrong way to do this. Simply observe and experience. Simply feel yourself smoothly breathing in and out, expanding your body in all directions. Notice the sensations in your skin, your muscles, your bones, and your internal organs as you observe your breath flow in and out. Expand. Become larger and lighter with each breath.

Continue the practice for as long as you like. When you begin to feel peaceful, calm, and tranquil, allow your mind to absorb the sensations while remaining keenly aware of how you are breathing.

It is natural for the mind to wander. If your mind becomes too active, or thoughts start to race, don't worry about it. Allow it to happen, gently focus your awareness on your breath as it softly expands and deflates your body. Feel each inhale nourish and soothe your body and mind. Feel each exhale release tension, toxins, and stale emotions.

When you are ready to end the practice, slowly to stretch the body, and gently roll to your side. Linger and rest. Be fully aware of your surroundings. Feel alert and present in your body. Slowly open your eyes and come to a sitting position. Pause and remember the pleasant sensations you experienced. Know that you can practice greater awareness of your breath at any time, and in any situation.

Present

Infinity is found in this one magnificent breath, now, in this one absolutely perfect moment.

*Breathe deep
and expand
your awareness.
Breathe deep
and broaden
your bandwidth.
Breathe deep
and heighten
your senses.*

More Breathing Awareness with Easy Movement

With practice, slow deep and steady breathing will become effortless and second nature. Coordinating breathing with simple movements can help you develop the ability to maintain sustained and heightened awareness of the breath.

This simple practice synchronizes slow, gentle physical movement, with the rhythm of your breath. This exercise can be done while sitting, standing, or lying down.

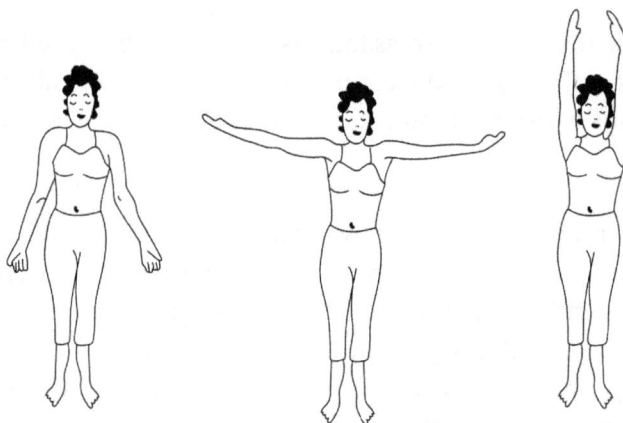

Begin by breathing in and out slowly. Relax your arms alongside your body.

As you slowly inhale, lift your arms up to shoulder height—either out to the side or in front of the body. Exhale as you lower the arms back down. Your arms should be alongside the body at the bottom of the exhale.

Repeat a few times coordinating the breath and movement of your arms. Keep them in sync. Arms are up at the peak of the inhale and arms are down at the end of the exhale. Be mindful of keeping your neck, shoulders, and chest relaxed.

Now make the movement larger and breath slower. Inhale as you slowly lift your arms up over your head. Make your inhale last until the arms are completely overhead. Exhale as you slowly lower your arms back down along your sides. Your exhalation should end as your arms are all the way down along your sides. Go slowly and make your movement match the pace of your breath.

Repeat this a few times experiencing the coordination of the movement and breathing. Relax and slow your breath and movement with every repetition. Continue to breathe and move increasingly slow. See how slowly you can go.

Now stretch. With a smooth, steady, even breath, extend your arms over the head. Bring your palms together and interlace your fingers. Turn your palms upward. Relax your shoulders and chest, and keep a slow, steady breath as your arms are stretched overhead. Try to soften your shoulders so that they slide down, instead of hunching up toward your ears. Relax as you breathe slowly with your arms stretched overhead.

Breathe softly and deeply for several moments while stretching your arms overhead. Keep your neck and shoulders soft, not tense. Relax and feel your abdomen expand as you inhale and contract as you exhale. You should feel your ribs, chest, and back expand and contract naturally and effortlessly. Stay relaxed and continue to soften your shoulders as you feel your lower belly and ribs expand and deflate with your breathing.

Happy

Inhale joy, peace, forgiveness, and infinite happiness. Feel these uplifting qualities penetrate into you and marinate in a sea of bliss. Exhale eternal love.

When you are ready to finish the practice, exhale as you lower your arms. Breathe naturally and spontaneously. Notice the relaxing yet energizing effects of the practice. Pause, rest, and enjoy your feelings and sensations.

Gross and Subtle Breath

Breath is both air and prana, gross and subtle. The gross, physical breath is simply the air moving into the body and out again. The experience of the gross breath is physical sensation. Air travels in and out. You can manipulate the gross breath by consciously controlling the movements of your body. Changing the rate of your breath, expanding and contracting muscles to increase and decrease air volume, and sending breath through either the nostrils or mouth are all examples of manipulating the gross, physical breath. Gross breathing is purely respiration. We use the gross physical breath in pranayama techniques, but gross breath alone is not pranayama. Pranayama requires mindfulness.

Pranayama teaches us to develop keen awareness of the subtle breath that lies within the gross breath. Subtle breath is prana. As we learn to observe the qualities of our breath, we begin to feel prana, the subtle breath within the physical. We begin our process of discovery with awareness of the ordinary, physical breath. But when our awareness evolves and we develop a higher awareness of the subtle movements supporting the breath, we expand our powers of perception. We expand our consciousness.

Try breathing through your mouth for a few moments, breathing athletically as if you are running up a flight of stairs. Pause and reflect on your experience of breathing athletically. Now try closing your eyes and slowly breathe through the nostrils with awareness. Observe the breath flow deeply into your body, expanding in all directions. Observe the breath softly flow out as your body gently deflates a little. Awareness of the subtle breath requires concentration. The mind relaxes and the experience of the subtle breath takes on an invisible psychic quality, and lighter, subtler frequency.

Gross and subtle breaths move in opposite directions. As the air travels down from the nostrils, into the throat, and deep into the lungs, you feel an uplifting, expansive sensation. While air travels down, prana is rising up. The expansive, energized, and uplifting sensation you feel on the inhale is the subtle breath, pure pranic energy. As you exhale, the physical air travels up and out, and you feel a relaxed sense of letting go, a subtle release, and gentle deflation. Air moves up and prana moves down as you exhale. Inhales pull fluid pranic energy up inside the nadi channels, while exhales release pranic energy downward through the body. As you breathe with conscious awareness, prana sweeps up and down throughout the vast network of nadis, smoothing out energy that may be congested, trapped, deficient, or excessive. The entire body receives balanced streams of pranic energy and operates harmoniously, efficiently, and vibrantly.

Magic

Breath flows down and in as prana expansively rises and lifts us up. Breath flows up and out as prana descends to ground and stabilize us.

Diaphragm Awareness

Many of us chronically hold tension in the respiratory diaphragm and solar plexus. When the diaphragm is weak, stressed, and constricted, we habitually breathe shallowly using only the upper parts of the lungs. Just like any other muscle structure in the body, when the diaphragm is tense and tight, the result is limited range of movement. The key to achieving big, full, rich, deep breathing is a pliable, elastic, and strong diaphragm. But most of us have never given a moment's notice to our diaphragm.

Rejuvenate

Send vital prana deep into your inner being and feel an unlimited source of renewable energy.

The respiratory diaphragm is a sheath of muscle and tissue separating the lower abdomen and the thoracic cavity—between the belly and the lungs. It is a dome-shaped membrane that attaches all around the circumference of your lower ribs. As you inhale the diaphragm contracts, flattens, and pulls downward toward the abdomen and outward against the lower rib structure. Air rushes in, the lungs inflate, the ribs blossom, and the lower belly swells. As you exhale, the diaphragm relaxes and forms a dome shape. The center of the diaphragm draws upward under the center of the ribcage, the lower ribs move inward as the lungs expire the breath up and out through the windpipe, mouth and nose.

The movement of a healthy diaphragm should be smooth and elastic. But unfortunately many of us have developed physical and emotional patterns that affect the health of the diaphragm and the quality of our breathing.

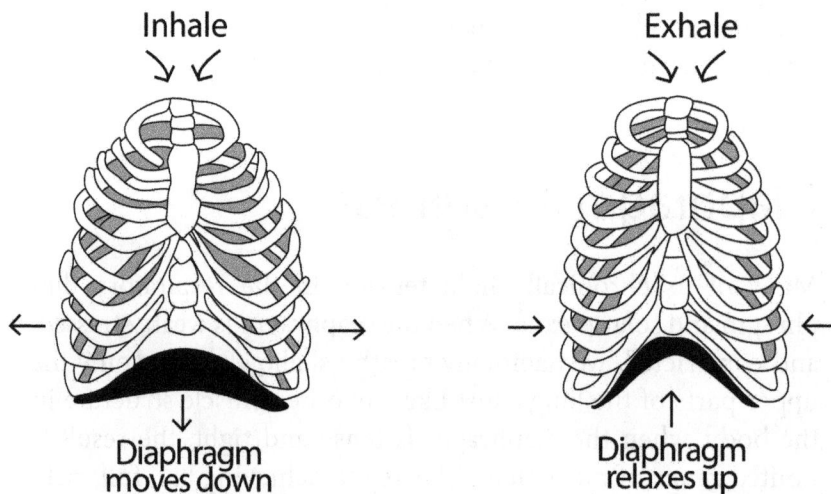

Inhale

Diaphragm
moves down

Exhale

Diaphragm
relaxes up

What Is Your Breathing Habit?

Blossom

*Make your belly
big and billowy
as you inhale,
relax deeply
as you exhale.
Blossom your
diaphragm.*

By now you probably have a pretty clear understanding that the belly should expand as you inhale and deflate as you exhale. But many of us have acquired habits and tendencies over the years that altered the pattern of our natural breath.

Chronic tension, anxiety, and scarcity of prana can lead to a shallow breathing pattern. Breath stays up high in the lungs, the diaphragm moves very little, and becomes weak and fatigued. Excessive emphasis on rock hard abs and a flat tummy can also lead to shallow breathing. Keeping the abs pulled in tight constricts the movement of the diaphragm, forcing respiration to the upper chest. A person that continually keeps the abdomen pulled in tight is usually tense, further restricting the respiratory volume. In addition to stress and anxiety disorders, over time shallow breathing may cause digestive and elimination problems. Strong, healthy abs are flexible. They can expand and billow fully then release and spring back. Flexible, strong abs and diaphragm work together to allow rich, full deep breathing.

Collapsed chest breathing can be a result of ongoing depression, illness, grief, or simply a sedentary lifestyle. Shoulders round forward, chest caves in, belly protrudes, and the head hangs heavy. The belly distends, and the muscle tone in the abs and diaphragm is flaccid and weak. Breath stays up high in short puffs, gasps, and wheezes. Circulation stagnates as prana congeals in the lower areas of the body, leading to numerous physical, mental, and emotional health issues.

Stress, competitive drive, and aggressive tendencies can lead to the very common habit of reverse breathing. In reverse breathing, as breath comes in during the inhale, the belly sucks in, the chest puffs out, the shoulders may rise, and the neck may stiffen.

Gifts

When you master your breath, life showers you with illuminations and the most luscious, spendid gifts that can only be realized through the soul.

On the exhale, the belly pushes out, the shoulders push back, and the chest my thrust forward. The diaphragm works in reverse to its natural pattern. A rigid, military-like posture often accompanies reverse breathing, holding the body in a stress pattern. Habitually cinching in the waistline can also lead to reverse breathing, never allowing the waist to expand and let go.

Constricted chest breathing is when the upper chest chronically tightens and the shoulders tend to hunch up. Fear, stress, and excessive use of computer keyboard can lead to constricted chest breathing. Increasingly, texting is also causing poor posture, leading to constricted chest breathing. The muscles of the upper back stiffen and the ribs immobilize. The diaphragm barely moves and very little air comes in and out. Patterns of anxiety and nervousness become habitual, keeping the body locked into the sympathetic nervous system response.

We can develop innumerable tendencies and habits that affect the way we breathe, but remember we all have the ability to control our breath, and to adopt vibrant, healthy breathing rhythms. Breathing reflects the state of your health, and your health reflects the way you breathe. Mindful, conscious breathing can lead to vibrant, radiant health, joyfulness, rejuvenation, and tranquility in your life. Awareness of your breathing patterns is the first and vital step.

Tune Into Your Diaphragm

*L*et's delve deeper into the inner processes of breathing. As you begin to explore the deeper movements of the respiratory diaphragm, you also begin to access subtler layers of your mental, emotional and spiritual being. The diaphragm lies deep inside the physical body. By learning to tune into our internal spaces, we learn to experience a profound connection to organic pranic energies. We feel the natural, harmonic rhythms and pulsations of our organs and bodily systems. As our connection to organic pranas strengthens, we begin to release unnecessary attachments to the external distractions in life that keep us held in states of stress, anxiety and limited awareness.

Relaxed and Strong Belly

The following practices are designed to help you focus on your belly and diaphragm. Some practices build strength and endurance, and others simply allow you to tune in, relax, and explore your breathing. As your diaphragm becomes stronger and more flexible you will breathe more deeply, and with greater fluidity. If you tend to hold stress in your abdomen, it may take some patience and practice to develop awareness and flexibility in the diaphragm. The most important thing is to take it easy, relax, and slowly let go. Remember, you were born breathing with a very flexible diaphragm and a very soft belly. It's natural. Let yourself be. Breath is a continual cycle, coming in and out like the tides. Your inner exploration is also a never-ending process of discovery, with infinite gifts of awareness and awakenings. Spend some quiet time with the practices you are drawn to.

Belly Breathing

Belly breathing, also called diaphragmatic breathing, or abdominal breathing, is gentle, easy and deeply relaxing. As we inhale, the diaphragm moves downward and our belly fills and expands. As we exhale, the diaphragm moves upwards, the belly softens inward, and the lungs deflate. In the belly breathing technique, we minimize the movement of our ribcage and maximize the movement of our diaphragm as we feel our belly inflate and deflate.

Begin by sitting up straight and tall or, if you like, practice belly breathing lying down on your back. Relax and begin to observe your natural, spontaneous breath. Feel at ease. Soften the skin on your face and feel your shoulders completely relax. Gently place your right hand on your belly just above the navel and place the left hand on your chest. Rest and breathe with your hands in this position.

As you breathe in and out, be aware of your right hand moving as your belly expands then deflates. Keep your chest still. Your left hand should not move. If you tend to bring breath into your chest, breathe more slowly and evenly, and focus your awareness on feeling your breath travel deep into the belly while relaxing your shoulders. Feel the hand on your belly rise and fall. Focus there. Simply breathe, relax, and observe.

Steady

Pranayama steadies the mind.

"When the breath wanders the mind also is unsteady. But when the breath is calmed the mind too will be still, and the yogi achieves long life. Therefore, one should learn to control the breath." Hatha Yoga Pradipika, 14th century CE

Tune Into Your Diaphragm

Savor

Savor the slow, sweet rhythm of your breath and marinate in the deep, still silence of your soul.

Continue for several more moments. Keep your ribs still as your abdomen expands and relaxes. Gradually slow down your breathing and bring in a bit more breath into your belly, keeping your ribs relaxed and still.

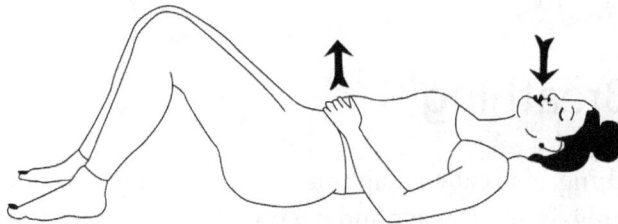

Belly Breathing Inhale

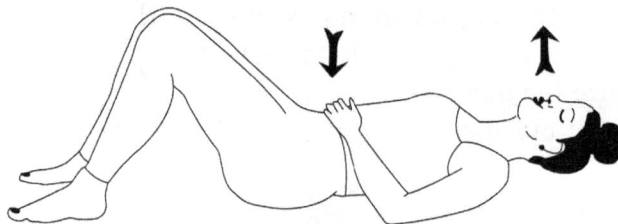

Belly Breathing Exhale

Now gently slide your left hand down to your belly so that both hands are resting on the abdomen. Touch your middle fingers together at your navel. Feel your entire abdominal area relax and expand as you inhale. You will feel your fingertips move away from each other as the belly expands. Never push the belly out, simply relax and allow the breath to flow in.

Allow your belly to deflate as you exhale. You will feel your hands move towards each other and middle fingers will touch as your breaths leaves your body. Remember to keep the belly as soft as possible. Really relax and let it go.

Continue for as long as you like. When you are ready to end the practice, take a few deep breaths and stretch your arms and legs. Become fully integrated and present in your body, then open your eyes. Pause, rest, and notice how you feel.

Relax

Simply breathe slow, deep and even. Relax and let go.

Belly Breathing Lying on Your Tummy

Relaxing the diaphragm for a smooth, even belly breath may not seem natural at first. Many of us are accustomed to feeling our breath up high in the chest, using the intercostal and chest muscles for breathing, and not so much the diaphragm. It may feel awkward to expand the belly instead of the chest. If you have been holding onto stress, or you habitually breathe inefficiently, changing your pattern to a deep, healthy belly breath can evoke feelings of anxiety. Lying on the abdomen to practice belly breathing can help. Practicing this way helps you naturally feel the movement of the belly. It is soothing, calming, grounding, and very comforting to feel the navel release into the supportive surface underneath you.

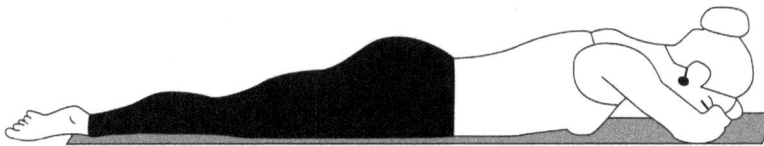

Tummy Breath Posture

To begin, lie on your tummy and rest your forehead on your folded arms. With the navel resting on the support beneath you, press into the arms to elevate your upper chest ever so slightly. You should be relaxed. If this causes stress in your shoulders, or if you are uncomfortable, try slightly adjusting the position

Empty

*Take a really,
really, really long
time to exhale.*

of your elbows and forearms, but keep the chest lifted. It may help to place a folded blanket or small pillow under the sternum for support. Your legs and feet should be relaxed, either together or separated, and your belly should be resting on the surface beneath you.

Close your eyes and feel your body relax. Let your internal organs feel heavy, and allow your entire abdominal region to relax and let go. Observe your breath, but don't try to change it in any way. Simply be. Breathe easily.

Bring your attention to your lower back. Feel the back softly expand as breath comes in, and feel your back deflate as you exhale. Feel your lower ribs expand and release as you breathe in and out. Feel the pressure of the belly swell into the surface below as you inhale. Feel the abdomen soften and deflate as you exhale. Feel, sense, and focus your awareness into your belly as you continue to breathe and relax. Linger like this for a little while, softening and focusing your attention on breathing in and out of the belly. Observe for as long as you are comfortable.

As you exhale, begin to consciously draw your navel up toward the spine and expel just a little bit more breath. Softly relax the belly and allow your breath to naturally flow in. Continue with extra awareness on sending your navel toward your spine at the end of the exhale.

As you breathe in, feel the skin and muscles around your lower back begin to ease and soften a bit more, yielding as the breath inflates and expands. Experience your lower back filling up, rising up, growing, expanding, releasing. Breathe in this way for a little while longer.

Inflate and expand your back and your belly as you inhale, like filling up a squishy balloon. Feel the pores of your skin soften and expand. While your back and belly are soft and widened, keep the sense of expansion as you exhale and draw your navel deeply toward your spine. Empty out every ounce of breath at the end of your exhale. Breathe in and out in this way until you feel comfortable with the sensations of deep, relaxed diaphragmatic breathing.

When you are ready to complete the practice, release your arms and lie comfortably on your tummy with your head turned to one side. Breathe naturally and spontaneously. Rest. Observe how you feel.

Bright

One day, while practicing pranayama, you will realize that you have eased into a deep state of meditation. Your breath will be smooth and easy, and your mind will be peaceful and clear. It will happen easily and effortlessly.

Watery Rubber Belly Breathing

Sometimes it can help to let your imagination go free to creatively visualize your breathing sensations. Oftentimes we think too much and overuse our intellect while trying to get a handle on the inner anatomy of the body. This practice encourages you to let go of the thinking mode, and joyfully imagine that your belly is a rubber balloon.

To begin, lie down on your back, bend your knees, and place the soles of your feet on the floor. Let your sacrum feel heavy and secure. Relax your belly. Really let it go soft.

Slowly breathe in through your nostrils as you imagine your lower belly is a water balloon filling up with water. Relax the belly. It will softly expand as more liquid breath fills in.

Overcome

Master your breath and you will master your thoughts, moods, and emotions.

Keep your face, throat, and shoulders soft and relaxed. Slowly deflate as you imagine the liquid breath pouring of your body. You may breathe out through your mouth if you like. As you exhale feel the entire surface of the front body gently melt down into the back. Keep exhaling until all of the liquid breath is gone.

Slowly fill the lower abdomen again, maintaining a fluid, liquid, gel-like quality of the breath. The belly expands in all directions. Slowly deflate until all of the liquid breath oozes completely out.

Continue for as long as you are comfortable. Then pause and notice how you feel.

For another sensation, try this in the bathtub or pool submerging your body up to the neck. The pressure of the water all around the body will help you feel the abdomen expand outward in all directions.

Soothing Embrace Breathing

This simple and beautiful practice helps you love and accept yourself, while nourishing your body and mind with prana.

Lie comfortably on your back and wrap your arms around yourself. Feel your lower ribs with your palms and fingers. Relax your shoulders. Just hug yourself. Soften the skin on your face. Relax your chest. Feel your ribcage expand and relax. Feel your folded arms elevate and lower as your belly swells and deflates. Breathe in love. Breathe out love. Inhale more love. Exhale more love.

Abdominal Control Breath

Bloom

Learn to breathe
deeply and fully,
and observe all
areas of your
life bloom into
the brilliant
expression of
your truest, most
sublime self.

While we want our bellies to expand during the inhale, it is important to maintain abdominal strength. The abdomen should expand as you inhale, but the lining of the abdominal wall should have integrity the entire time. This breath helps you learn to expand as you inhale while maintaining relaxed control of the abdomen.

Sit up nice and tall, either in an easy cross-legged position, or in a chair with the feet firmly placed on the ground. Take a few slow, deep and easy breaths. Relax the shoulders and face. Place the left hand on your lower belly, just under the navel, and the right hand just above the navel. Take a big breath in and then expel all of the breath out. Feel the belly draw back to the spine as the air leaves. Press your palms slightly against the abdomen as you breathe in. The belly will press against your palms. Feel the breath fill into the front, sides, and back of the abdominal wall. Keep a gentle, but firm, pressure of your palms on the belly, and feel your abdomen expand a bit as it presses into the palms. Feel the sides and back of the abdomen expand as breath comes in. The belly deflates back to the spine as you breathe out.

Repeat for several minutes. When you are ready to end the practice, lower your hands and take a few deep, full breaths. Begin to breathe spontaneously and naturally. Pause, rest, and notice how you feel.

Diaphragm Strengthening Breath

This practice builds strength of the abdominal wall and stamina in and around the diaphragm. Sit up nice and tall, or lie down on your back, on a firm surface. Bend your elbows and grasp your torso just underneath the lowest rib with your palms wide, thumbs toward your back, and fingers spread. Inhale and gently press in on your lower ribs as they expand. Keep a firm, but not extreme, pressure for the diaphragm to press out against. Relax the pressure as you exhale. Take slow, full breaths, and exert a steady pressure with your hands. Your diaphragm will need to strengthen to expand and push the lower ribs open. Feel your lower ribs expand against the pressure of your hands. Breathe slowly, deeply, and smoothly.

Release the practice after a short while. Rest. Breathe smoothly and spontaneously. Notice how you feel.

Belly Breathing with Abdominal Weight

It is important to relax and also to develop deep inner strength in the abdominal region. Just like any muscle in your body, extended periods of inactivity will weaken the diaphragm and abdominal support structures.

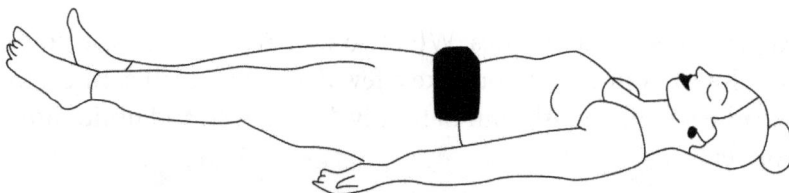

Belly Breathing with Weight

Resting a light weight on the lower abdomen while practicing belly breathing is a soothing, grounding, and relaxing way to bring more attention into the belly while strengthening the diaphragm and abdominal muscles. In a yoga studio, it is common to use a sandbag for this purpose, but at home you may use an open heavy book, bags of rice, or similarly weighted item that will balance on your belly.

Begin by lying comfortably on your back on the floor, or other firm surface. Lying on a soft bed or sofa will not provide adequate support for your spine and back ribs. You may want to place a small support behind the knees. Be relaxed and comfortable.

Become aware of the natural, spontaneous breath until you breathe smoothly and easily. Relax the belly and feel it become elastic, inflating as you inhale. Feel your belly relax and deflate on the exhalation. Keep the breath slow, smooth, deep, and even.

When you have established a smooth, steady and relaxed breath, place the weight (sandbag, book etc.) on the belly at the navel, or slightly above. Do not place the weight below the navel near the pubic bone. The pressure of the weight will heighten your awareness of the abdomen. As you slowly breathe in and out, the weight will rise as the abdomen swells and lower as the abdomen deflates. Do not try to push into the weight, simply breathe in and out. Your abdominal muscles and diaphragm will strengthen as they work to expand with the added resistance of the weight.

Relax completely and breathe smoothly, deeply, and evenly. The weight will encourage a more rapid exhalation and slower inhalation, so try to maintain a smooth and steady rhythm.

Keep breathing in this way for a little while. If you begin to feel fatigued or weak, stop the practice and rest. When you feel ready to close the practice, gently remove the weight, and breathe naturally. Take some time to notice how you feel.

Glow

Consciously bring your breath in very slowly. Breathe in as long and deep and relaxed as you can. Send it gently out as slowly and as fully as you can.

Tune Into Your Diaphragm

*Love the shape
of your belly.
Softness and a
little belly fat
is ok. Really.
Be strong,
be happy, be
comfortable, and
be healthy. Just
be and breathe.
Appreciate,
celebrate and
truly love your
body.*

Diaphragm Expansion Breath

In this practice, we use the help of an elastic exercise band, or stretchy bandage wrap, to apply resistance for the diaphragm to push against. It is a strengthening practice that will build up endurance and vitality, and will help you feel the movements of the diaphragm.

Stretch an elastic exercise band or bandage wrap slightly below your lower ribs. Adjust the tension so it's not too slack or too tight. You want just enough tension and resistance to feel movement in your midsection and diaphragm.

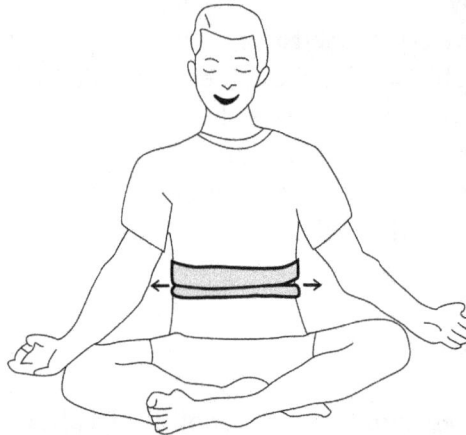

Diaphragm Strengthing with Elastic Band

Sit up tall with a straight spine. Breathe slowly, keeping your chest still and your belly soft. Try to feel the band securely and evenly as you breathe. As you inhale, feel resistance as your diaphragm pushes outward. Feel the elastic band expand. As you deflate on the exhale, feel the tension of the band slacken.

Continue breathing and feeling into this for several moments. Explore a little while, then relax and rest before starting the practice again. A little goes a long way. You are working and building muscle tone. Try not to fatigue the diaphragm and intercostal muscles. It is best to work gently over time.

When you are ready to end the practice, gently release the band, stretch, move, and breathe normally. Pause, rest, and notice how you feel.

Back Breathing

This breathing practice allows you to feel the full expansion of diaphragm, lungs, and back ribs. It is excellent for releasing tension. Most of us spend all of our awareness in the front body and very little in the back body. The front body is where we place our attention on moving forward into the future. Our mind moves from thought to thought, propelling us on to the next thing, and anticipating events yet to come. We tend to neglect our back body when we breathe, and most of us hold stress in the back. When we breathe, we easily feel the front of the body expand, but the back often remains stiff and tight. In this practice, we learn to use the front, sides, and back of the body when we breathe. We connect to the sensation of opening, broadening, and expanding our back body. Our back relaxes and more breath and prana can expand into the back regions. Our mind and body can experience a "letting go" of anxiety, and we feel fully present in the moment of breath.

Tune Into Your Diaphragm

Conscious

Throughout the day, become fully conscious of your breath. Observe how your breath fluctuates as you experience a diverse palette of thoughts, activities, and emotions.

This practice is gentle and relaxing. As you let go of stress your back ribs and torso can become more pliable. Your diaphragm will exert pressure into the lower back ribs and they will begin to yield. Your breathing will become slower, deeper, and more efficient. Your back body will soften.

Begin by lying down on your back, with knees bent and soles of feet on the surface below. It's best to use a padded, but firm surface; such as a mat or blanket on the floor. Slowly breathe in and feel where the back body is making contact with the surface below you. Make any adjustments to your hips and pelvis to reduce arching your lower back. Feel the skin on your back begin to soften.

Breathe slowly, deeply, and evenly. Softly inhale and feel more of your back body spread and press into the floor. Feel the entire surface of your back expand and become heavier. Perceive the skin on your back soften even more. Relax and exhale. Breathe in slowly and deeply, and allow the entire back surface to spread wider and feel heavier as it melts into the surface beneath you. Relax deeply and exhale. Continue as long as you like.

You may also practice back breathing while sitting up against a firm surface. Sit up straight where you can feel the back surface of your body gently press against the back of a chair, or any firm surface; such as a wall or headboard of your bed. You may place a small pillow or folded towel in the curve of the lower back so that you can feel the entire surface of your back press against a surface.

As you slowly and deeply inhale, feel your body widen. Soften the skin of your back and feel the surface of your back body gently press and expand across the firm surface of the support behind you. Relax and feel the mid back press into the firm surface.

Breathe deeply. Relax a bit more on the exhale and feel the lower back begin to press into the surface behind you. Feel the skin on the back, shoulders, and neck soften and lengthen.

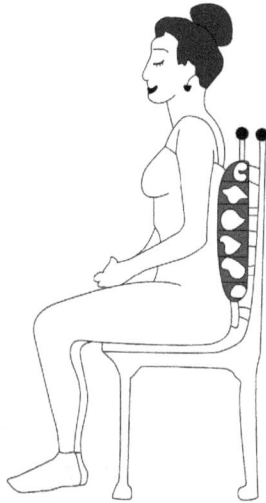

Seated Back Breathing

Slowly repeat as many times as you like, relaxing and expanding the back body on the inhale, and slightly elongating the spine on the exhale.

Back breathing is a nice practice to do in the car while stopped at a light or stopped in traffic. You can hold the steering wheel to help press the lower and mid-back into the seat, while you feel your back ribs expand.

Cherish

Breathe into the heart of love and cherish the beautiful power of deep intimacy that dwells within every breath.

Back Breathing with a Partner

Breathing with a partner is a lovely way to practice back breathing. Allowing your breath and subtle movements to harmonize with another person is healing, therapeutic, and pleasant.

Sit with your partner, back to back. Adjust your postures, and be comfortable. It's a good idea to sit up on a folded blanket or a pillow to elevate your hips. You may link elbows with one another or simply allow your arms to rest in your laps or sides.

Simple

Want to reduce anxiety? Simply make your exhale last longer than your inhale.

Begin to breathe slowly, feeling your back bodies press against one another. Communicate nonverbally as you increase the surface of your backs connecting with one another. Breathe together slowly. Soften into each other. Try not to push each other out of balance, but make every movement very subtle and in harmony with your partner.

Breathe with each other for as long as you like, experiencing harmony and intimacy. This feels so nice, you won't want to stop!

Gentle Sacrum Rocking Breath

We spend most of our waking awareness directed toward the front of our bodies. It's important to expand our ability to pay conscious attention to the sensations, feelings, and movements occurring in our back body. This gentle sacrum rocking breath relaxes the lower back and stimulates sensory awareness of the sacral region while softly synchronizing breath and movement.

Begin by lying down on your back. Bend your knees and place the soles of your feet on the surface beneath you. Your arms may rest on the surface beneath you, extended to the sides—like cactus arms with the palms facing upward, or simply extended overhead. Breathe slowly and relax.

Become aware of the sacrum, the flat bony structure at the base of your spine. Slowly begin to move the hips, tracing the outline of the sacrum on the surface below you. Roll around the edges of the sacrum in one direction for a few moments, then reverse. Eventually, come to a still point and rest. Notice any feelings and sensations.

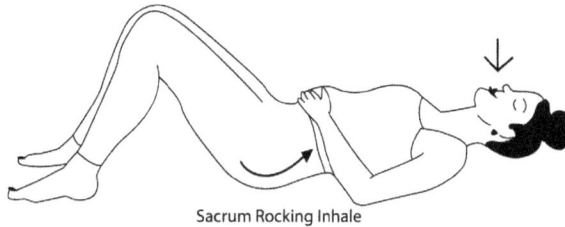
Sacrum Rocking Inhale

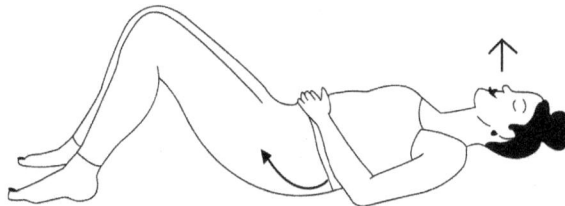
Sacrum Rocking Exhale

Next begin to slowly inhale as you press the lower edge of the sacrum, nearest the tail bone, into the surface beneath you. The upper edge will lift. As you slowly exhale, rock the sacrum so that the top edge presses into the surface beneath you. Inhale as the tail bone side presses down, exhale as the top edge presses down. Feel your navel soften, widen, and expand as you inhale. Feel your navel pull in, contracting toward the spine as you breathe out. Keep the movement and breath very slow and steady. Develop a very slow and relaxed rhythm.

Continue for as long as you like. When you are complete with the practice, pull your knees up into your chest and give yourself a hug. Then stretch the legs out and reach the arms overhead. Relax and notice how you feel.

*The breath is
an invisible link
between the
layer of the body
and the layer of
the mind.*

Yogi Breath or Three-Part Breath: Dirga Pranayama

In Sanskrit, dirga pranayama means complete breath. This breath technique fills up the lower belly, mid chest, then upper chest in one slow and fluid inhale. The exhale flows in reverse, emptying the upper chest, mid chest, then lower abdomen. Yogi breath maximizes the amount of oxygen you bring in to your body and increases prana. It energizes and purifies our bodies on a cellular level, clears and calms the mind, and allows us to focus on the present moment. This breath is very easy to learn and forms the foundation for more advanced breathing techniques. Dirga pranayama is often used for stress management and is a very effective way to begin a meditation practice.

You can practice either sitting or lying down. Begin by observing your natural breath. Breathe slowly, evenly and deeply. Try to make your breath silent and smooth as it flows in and out of your body. Relax. Keep your face soft, and neck and shoulders fully relaxed.

Bring your breath slowly in as you soften and fill up the lower belly. When the belly becomes full, begin to fill up the ribs and chest, expanding outward and upward. When the chest and ribs are filled completely, continue to relax and bring in a bit more air into the upper chest. You will feel your collarbones, back of your neck, and shoulders rise up very slightly. Bring in as much air as possible without tensing up. Pause briefly at the top of the inhale.

As you begin to exhale, make a smooth transition with no gasping or catching. Smoothly and gently allow the breath to release from the upper clavicle region, chest and ribs, then the lower belly.

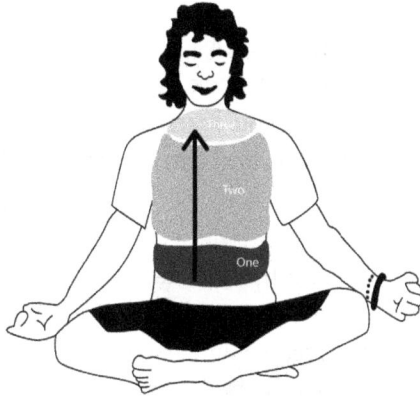

Three Part Breath

Begin softly and easily. Gradually let the breath deepen. Remain comfortable and relaxed throughout the entire practice. Repeat. Smoothly breathe in and fill up the lower belly, then chest, then collar bones, and back of the neck all in one smooth, fluid breath. Keep the breath gentle and even. Do not force.

Imagine a liquid quality to your breath, like flowing water pouring from a pitcher, naturally filling up the abdomen, then ribs, then upper chest—filling up to full capacity. Pause just briefly at the top, keeping your face, shoulders, and neck relaxed. Then seamlessly release your breath in a smooth, even stream moving from the collarbones, chest, and then belly.

As the breath begins to leave the belly area, you may actively pull in the abdomen, sending your navel back toward the spine. This will help the breath move up and out of the body. Practice for several minutes then pause and rest. Notice how you feel.

Tune Into Your Diaphragm

Release

Let go of all tension in your chest, neck and throat to encourage the rich, full expansion of breath.

More Three-Part Breath

For most people beginning to learn yogi breathing, the upper chest breath portion of the technique is the most difficult to master. Most of us hold chronic tension in the neck and shoulders, and it may feel unnatural at first to release and soften the upper chest, shoulders, and back of neck. With practice, this tension will naturally melt away as you learn to gently relax the upper chest, collarbones, shoulders, and throat as breath fills into these higher regions.

If you find yourself tensing up and using effort to fill the upper chest, it may help to practice yogi breathing while comfortably lying down. In this practice, we will also use our hands to feel the sequence of movements in the belly, ribs, and chest.

Begin by breathing into the lower belly and ribs. Close your eyes. Relax your face and body, and breathe naturally through your nose.

Place your left hand on your lower belly, just below your navel, and place your right hand on the outer right edge of your rib cage, so you can feel your side ribs expand and relax.

As you inhale, feel your belly expand, then feel your ribs expand.

As you exhale, feel your ribs deflate, then your belly. Exhale completely as you press your palm very gently on your abdomen to help release your breath. Do this a few times until it begins to feel easy and natural.

Next, relax your right hand and rest it alongside your body. Slide your left hand to your chest, just below your collarbone. As you slowly inhale, fill up the belly, then the mid chest, and finally the upper chest. Feel your collarbones swell into your left palm as your chest broadens and slightly rises.

Fully exhale, first from the upper chest, then mid chest. As your breath leaves the lower abdomen, feel your navel descend into the abdominal cavity toward your spine.

Relax and continue yogi breathing with both arms alongside your body. As you inhale, your belly lifts, then your ribs expand, and your chest rises all the way up to the collarbones. As you exhale, your collarbones release, your chest drops, your ribs deflate, and your belly softens and lowers. Continue at your own pace for as long as you feel comfortable.

When you are ready to end the practice, breathe naturally and spontaneously. Pause, rest, and be aware of how you feel.

The Art and Action
of Moving Prana

*M*astering the flow of prana requires conscious attention, skill, applied technique and artistry. Developing mastery also requires time and practice. Learning to direct the flow of prana can be compared to learning to play a musical instrument. First, you master basic notes, then simple tunes, and eventually more complex musical compositions. Your music may sound primitive and unpolished at first, but with practice your sound becomes clear and polished. Mastering the flow of prana through pranayama will lead you to great heights of conscious awareness. Let's take a look at some foundational components.

Moving Prana

We can learn to use awareness, our breathing, and physical mechanics to consciously direct the flow of our vital energy, our prana. When we consciously channel our prana, we send healing, vibrant energy into specific areas of our body by opening and purifying specific nadis.

Many pranayama practices use a technique called bandha (BUN-duh) to help direct the flow of our prana. The word bandha means to lock, hold, or tighten. Three commonly used bandhas are the root lock, abdominal lock, and throat lock. Some pranayama techniques also utilize specific rhythmic breathing patterns, or breathing retention, to control the flow of prana. In more advanced techniques, bandhas are applied while holding the breath in, and also while pausing the breath after exhalation.

Root Lock: Mula Bandha

Mula (MOO-luh) means root or base, and bandha means lock. The root lock provides a secure base so that prana does not seep out of the body at the bottom, but can instead begin to rise expansively up and out of the root to enliven and energize all layers of your body. We activate mula bandha by engaging, energizing, and drawing up the pelvic floor, the perineum.

Mula bandha helps amplify and recirculate prana to revitalize and regenerate our life-supporting energies. It may help to think of the root lock as a seal at the base of your body keeping the contents of your subtle energy body intact and secure, much like the bottom of a pot or the base of bowl. You can imagine that by activating mula bandha, a seal is created at the base of your body, securely established at the root of your torso between the anus and urethra. When this seal is created, prana can increase and strengthen, and does not dissipate, or leak out from the body. When mula bandha is applied, concentrated nerve complexes in the pelvic area are stimulated, amplifying vital pranic energies that course upward through the nadis and energy centers at the chakra points.

Learning to consciously apply the root lock will enhance your breathing practices. Physically, it is similar to the women's Kegel exercise, or the action of stopping the flow of urine midstream,

Oneness

Through slow, calm, deep and steady breathing, the mind can achieve a state where separation merges into oneness.

but mula bandha is not a tight gripping or strong compression. It is more energetic than physical, like a strong magnetic current pulling up, prompting an energetic lift of prana.

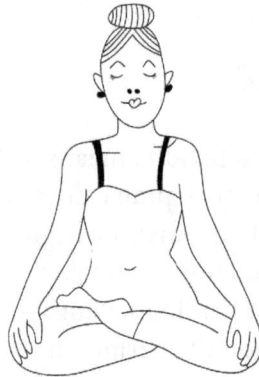

To engage mula bandha, sit in a comfortable posture where the hips are supported and stable. Breathe naturally and slowly. Begin by simply and lightly contracting the pelvic floor and drawing it upward. Keep the lifting sensation engaged for a little while, then gently release. Repeat several times, lift up the perineum, pause for a brief time, and relax fully. Contract the pelvic floor and let it go. You will begin to strengthen the pelvic floor, and become more aware of the energetic sensations with practice.

Relaxed Posture

Now try relaxing the pelvic floor and breathing softly. Use inner awareness to locate a point in the perineum between the anus and the urethra that feels a bit brighter and more energetic than the surrounding area. Keep the anus relaxed, and draw up only this concentrated point of heightened sensation. Keep the surrounding areas relaxed. Pause briefly, then release. Repeat several times. Rest for a good while before practicing another round. It is important to take this practice in short segments so the system does not fatigue or become over-stimulated.

Try mula bandha with breath retention, antara kumbhaka. Sit comfortably and breathe slowly. Begin to sense the energetic point in the perineum. Simultaneously, be aware of the eyebrow center, ajna chakra. As you breathe in, begin to contract mula bandha slowly and steadily as you feel the breath rise up to ajna chakra. Synchronize your awareness of mula bandha and the breath rising up to ajna chakra. Retain the breath in while holding mula bandha and concentrating on the eyebrow center. Make sure the rest of the body is relaxed. As you relax, exhale slowly and be aware of prana moving down from the eyebrow center to the root. Try it again. Breathe in from the root to the eyebrow center as you draw in mula bandha. Increase the sensation as the breath is held in. Relax and flow the breath out from the eyebrow center to the root.

Now try mula bandha while pausing and holding the breath out after the exhale. Inhale deeply then exhale all of the breath out. Hold breath out for 5 seconds as you gently contract mula bandha. Feel the energetic and physical lift. The navel point will naturally draw in a bit. Slightly relax the contraction as you inhale. Repeat several times. As your ability to hold the breath out develops, gradually lengthen the duration of mula bandha. Become more aware of mula bandha by gently and rhythmically pulsing the contraction, without allowing it to fully release.

You can engage mula bandha anytime, anywhere, however be gentle and build slowly over time. Remember, it takes time and lots of practice to develop mastery of the mula bandha technique. Be patient, explore, enjoy the practice, and learn to experience subtle effects over time.

Abdominal Lock: Uddiyana Bandha

Uddiyana (OO-dee-ah-nah) means to fly up or rise up, and bandha means lock. Uddiyana bandha activates the navel center, circulating fresh vital prana inward and upward. The practice of uddiyana bandha is highly beneficial physically, emotionally,

Glide

Feel your belly button soften and glide out as you inhale and smoothly glide back in as you exhale.

The Art and Action of Moving Prana

Magnetize

Pulsate and activate your navel center. Charge it up and feel your inner magnetism.

and energetically. The abdominal organs are massaged, revitalized, and squeezed like sponges, eliminating toxins and stagnation. All the internal organs are toned and strengthened. Highly concentrated prana in the navel center and the solar plexus, are activated and distributed throughout the body. Uddiyana bandha stabilizes the nervous system, strengthens circulation and digestion, and creates feelings of strength, empowerment, and confidence.

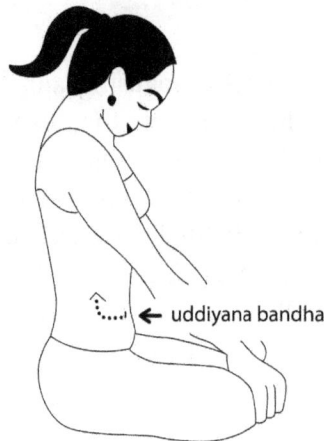

← uddiyana bandha

To begin, first exhale all of your breath out. With the breath held out, pull your navel back toward your spine and upward toward the back ribs. This causes the diaphragm to lift up. Then completely soften the belly, inhale, and relax. Exhale, pull the navel up and in, relax the belly then inhale. Repeat several times, then rest.

When practicing uddiyana bandha, try to isolate your abdomen, just as in the belly breathing techniques. It's important to keep your shoulders, neck, and face relaxed. Remember you want your energy to rise up, so reducing tension in your upper body will help vital prana flow up smoothly and permeate deeply into your chest, shoulders, neck, and head.

It may also help to first gently activate mula bandha before you pull the navel in. You will notice that a gentle sensation of uddiyana bandha naturally occurs as you engage the root lock. When you find this awareness, simply direct more attention to the navel area and draw it further inward and upward.

Be gentle, and try not to tense up the belly area. With practice, the abdominal muscles will strengthen and become more flexible, and uddiyana bandha will feel easy and natural. You will feel more sensation around the navel and develop greater awareness and ability to increase pranic energy there.

Go slowly, and when you are learning to engage uddiyana bandha, limit your practice sessions to just a few minutes at a time. Allow yourself plenty of time to fully relax and rest between practices. Be patient, and build strength and concentration over time.

Infinite

Breath exists on all planes of manifestation.

Throat Lock: Jalandhara Bandha

Jalandhara (JAH-lan-dhah-ruh) means flowing or throat, and bandha means lock. The throat lock helps expand the flow of prana, especially to the upper back, neck, and head. Jalandhara bandha stretches the back of the neck, releases blockages in the upper spine to the base of the skull, and keeps the head and upper body in proper alignment for optimal flow of prana. You should practice pranayama with some degree of jalandhara bandha, even if only a slight engagement. Jalandhara bandha elicits a parasympathetic response because it directly stimulates the vagus nerve where it nears the surface of the pharynx. Without jalandhara bandha, some pranayamas can place excess constriction in the neck and throat, pressure may accumulate in the upper torso and

The Art and Action of Moving Prana

head, and heart rate and blood pressure can elevate. A very gentle jalandhara bandha during all relaxing and soothing pranayamas will enhance the tranquil and peaceful effects.

To begin, sit in a comfortable, stable posture with a straight spine. Exhale all of the breath out, and then breathe in. As the breath flows in, lift the chest up so that the top of the sternum rises toward the chin. Pull the chin back to elongate the back of the neck. Try not to lower the chin down to the chest so much that the back rounds, rather breathe into the upper chest so that the chest inflates and rises up to meet the chin. Then draw the chin back. You will need to relax and soften the sternum and shoulders to do this. Roll the shoulders back and slide the shoulder blades downward toward the back ribs. This requires just a bit of flexibility in the upper back, which will begin to develop naturally over time. Eventually, the chin may draw back and appear to nestle into the throat pit as the sternum expands and rises up.

Inhale as slowly as you can while drawing your chin back, lifting your sternum and sliding your shoulder blades downward toward your back ribs. Pause at the very top of the inhale with jalandhara engaged. Release the throat lock and softly, slowly exhale. Inhale, lift the sternum as the chin pulls back toward the throat pit and back of neck elongates. Relax, release, and exhale. Repeat a few more times, making sure you rest a good amount of time in between.

Be gentle. Take it slowly and lightly. Never force or strain. Remember, it takes lots time and practice to master these techniques. Slow, steady progress, just a little at a time, is best. Make sure you rest fully in between practices.

Great Lock: Maha Bandha

Maha means great or highest. Maha bandha is the application of the root, abdominal, and throat locks at the same time. It provides all of the benefits of mula, uddiyana, and jalandhara bandhas. Maha bandha is a supreme practice highly regarded by yogis for thousands of years due to its vast benefits. Proper practice regulates the endocrine system, activates the pineal gland, stimulates the vagus nerve, slows the aging process, and rejuvenates all the systems.

It is important to be proficient in mula, uddiyana, and jalandhara bandhas before practicing maha bandha. If you feel ready to try it, begin sitting in a stable position with the hips and legs secure and grounded. Sitting cross-legged in a yoga pose, such as sukhasana or lotus, is recommended.

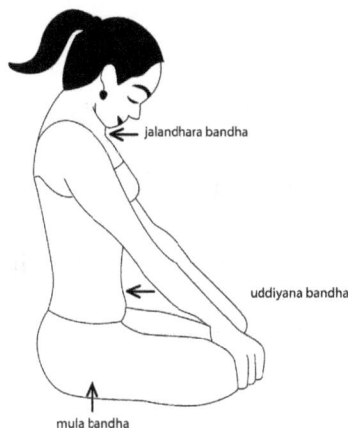

Begin by breathing slowly, deeply and evenly. Take a big, deep breath in through the nose, and quickly expel all of the breath out as you exhale through the mouth. Close your lips and hold your breath out. Apply jalandhara bandha, then uddiyana bandha,

Invite

Invite breath in. Let it stay awhile. Enjoy its company. Let your joy linger long after the breath travels on.

and then mula bandha. Hold as long as comfortable, without straining or forcing. Slowly release mula bandha, then uddiyana bandha, then jalandhara bandha, and finally inhale slowly.

Pause, relax, and breathe naturally before beginning another round. Exhale all the breath out, apply jalandhara, then uddiyana, and then mula bandha. Don't strain. Relax and release mula, then uddiyana then jalandhara bandha, and inhale.

Maha bandha is a very powerful practice. Take it easy and practice only a few rounds. Don't overdo it and never ever strain. It takes time and practice to become proficient, and you do not want to develop incorrect or sloppy habits. It is important to be gentle. Prana flowing through the network of nadis can become easily disturbed and unbalanced if an aggressive or forceful pressure is applied. Remember, less is more. A little goes a very long way. Be patient and make progress slowly.

Inhale, Exhale, Pause: Puraka, Rechaka, Kumbhaka

There are four parts of the breath to explore in pranayama: inhalation, puraka (POO-ra-kuh); retaining the breath in, antara kumbhaka (AN-ta-ruh) (KOOM-bha-kuh); exhalation, rechaka (REH-chuh-kuh); and suspending the breath out, bahya kumbhaka (BHY-uh) (KOOM-bha-kuh).

Puraka is the inspiration, the inhale. Breath flowing into your body is expansive, nourishing, and enlivening. Our in-breath draws in fresh oxygen and vital universal prana into our body to nourish every aspect of our lives. Inhaling is active, uplifting, and heating. Puraka unites the cosmic infinite with the finite.

Rechaka is the expiration, the exhale. Breath flowing out of our body is cleansing, detoxifying, and calming. Our out-breath expels carbon dioxide and toxic residues. Exhaling is soothing, relaxing, and cooling. Rechaka releases the individual self into the infinite cosmic whole.

Kumbhaka is the neutral steady state between inspiration and expiration. It is suspension, tranquility, and quietude. Kumbhaka should be comfortable. If there is stress or strain, it is not kumbhaka. Suspension of breath is bliss, not effort. The senses withdraw into the placid stillness between the motions of breathing in and breathing out. The mind is silenced in the undisturbed, soundless space of no breath at all. Kumbhaka comes from the root word kund, meaning to contain, or the container. Kumbhaka contains the breath in infinite stillness. Vedic teachings place a great deal of importance on kumbhaka, and some sources define the entire practice of pranayama as kumbhaka.

Antara kumbhaka is the vast quiescence of breath contained with the realms of the physical body. Breath is held in. The internal spaces of the body expand into infinity. Bahya kumbhaka is perfect oneness with the universal infinite cosmos beyond the physical body. Breath is held out. A third kumbhaka, kevala (KHE-vuh-luh), is a spontaneous, naturally occurring, blissful state of breath suspension. Kevala kumbhaka arises organically and is very similar to the deep state of inner bliss, samadhi (sa-MAH-dhee), as all layers of the mind and body merge into oneness with the infinite cosmos.

Establish an Internal Rhythm

We have all experienced holding our breath. It's a natural exploration. Kids play to see how long they can hold their breath,
try to make it from one end of the swimming pool to the other
underwater without surfacing, and threaten to hold breath for-
ever to punish a parent or sibling. Retaining the breath in traditional pranayama, however, is conferred great respect and taught
with the highest integrity, gentleness, and precious care. Breath
retention trains our bodies to be calm as carbon dioxide levels rise in our bloodstream, triggering our innate reflex to take
in fresh oxygen. Natural anxieties resulting from the "fight or
flight" sympathetic nervous system response will present a challenge to remain calm. You should aim for a steady rhythm and
equanimity of mind, emotion, and breathing during all phases
of the breath cycle. Great care is required to ensure prana travels
throughout the body's delicate system of nadis with balanced,
precisely appropriate amounts of pressure, velocity, and ampli-
tude. We never want to apply too much force or linger too long
past the point of steady control.

A steady rhythm will help you maintain stable and calm when
practicing pranayama with breath retention. You should never
hold your breath so long that you need to gasp or roughly expel.
The transitions between inspiration and expiration should be
silky smooth—no catching, gasping, or abrupt segues. Your
breath should flow softly and smoothly into the body. Face,
throat, shoulders, chest, and back should remain soft and relaxed
as the breath is retained. Very subtly, almost imperceptibly, the
breath should begin to flow out until it is completely absent from
the body. Suspend lightly and gently with no breath. The body
and mind remain fully relaxed as a fresh wave of breath stream
flows into the body.

When you are beginning a kumbhaka practice, you may have a natural tendency to speed up your count as feelings of anxiety begin to arise. Try your best to maintain a constant, steady rhythm.

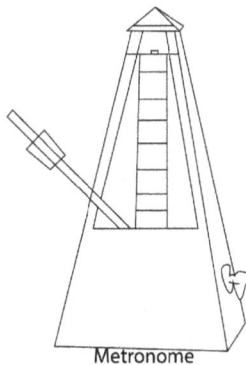

Metronome

It may be helpful to use a metronome, metronome app, or click track beat to emit an audible, measured, steady beat. Playing a soothing, cadenced mantra recording in the background can also be helpful in maintaining a constant, steady beat.

Easy, Soothing Four-Part Breath

In this easy pranayama, we begin breathing steadily to a measured rhythm. Inhale, retention in, exhale, and holding out are all of equal duration. When all parts of the breath are equal in duration, it is called same breath, sama vritti (SAH-mah) (VRIT-hee) pranayama. Sama means same and vritti is a movement or fluctuation of energy. Puraka, antara kumbhaka, rechaka, and bahya kumbhaka are equal.

Scope

Pranayama involves dimensions of space, time, and beyond. Approach pranayama practice as an explorer of the vast and infinite.

Begin by finding a comfortable posture. Sitting or lying down is fine, just be comfortable. Begin slow, deep and even breathing. Focus on the breath coming into and out of the nostrils. Begin ujjayi breathing. Relax and find a rhythm. It may be helpful to listen to a metronome beat.

Let's begin with the count of three. Breathe in three counts. Hold three counts. Exhale three counts. Hold out three counts. Breathe in three. Hold three. Breathe out three. Hold out three. Feel steady and comfortable. Continue to practice four-part breathing to the count of three for several moments.

Rhythm and concentration are more important than length of breath and holds. If you feel steady and focused and relaxed, then you may increase the count to four. Puraka four counts. Antara kumbhaka four counts. Rechaka four counts. Bahya kumbhaka four counts. Stay with this rhythm for several minutes. Breathe in four, hold four, breathe out four, and hold out four. Feel the transitions. Make them gentle and smooth with no rough edges.

You may end the practice, or choose to deepen your concentration and increase the count to five. Stay with the beat of five for several minutes. Stop and rest at any time. Keep an even, slow and smooth flow. The transitions should be effortless.

If you continue to the count of six, pay increased attention to deepening your concentration. Be aware of the steady flow of breath and the fluid transitions between phases. Keep it steady. Notice if tension builds in the upper chest on the inhale and inward retention. Notice if your energy drops as you begin to hold the breath out. Maintain balance and equanimity. Don't compromise, simply go back to a lower count until you feel balance and ease.

As you are ready to complete the practice, release the count. Breathe spontaneously and naturally. Be aware of your surroundings. Notice all sensations in your body, and observe the state of your mind. Notice how you feel. Pause, rest, and be still for a good while before continuing with other activities.

Infinite Spaciousness of Breath

As we fine-tune our awareness of breath, we begin to feel and experience breathing in brand new ways. New dimensions and insights emerge as the spectrum of our conscious awareness expands. We begin to sharpen our awareness, finely tune our perceptions and notice subtleties in our breath. The quality of space in our breath is something we naturally tune in to as our pranayama practice evolves and deepens over time.

Discerning if the breath is inside or outside of the body is one of the first spatial qualities we perceive in the early stages of pranayama practice. We consciously explore bringing the breath in and sending it out. We begin to broaden our awareness of the subtler qualities of the breath. How does the breath feel? Is it thin and weak, or full and robust? Is it dense or light?

We explore spaciousness when we observe and control the length of the breath. Try taking in a very long, deep breath. Compare the space of the breath at the beginning, middle, and end of the inhale. Did the breath space become more compact, squeezed and compressed at the end? Take another long, deep breath and try to keep a steady stream the entire duration of the inhale. Did your neck, shoulders, chest, and back relax toward the end of the inhale as you tried to keep the breath space constant and full?

The Art and Action of Moving Prana

Limitless

As you richly inhale, sense that you are receiving energy from a pure, eternal source of perfect divinity. Feel every cell and atom in your body swell with abundant, fresh, pure, vital prana. Breathe out far and deep into the limitless, infinite cosmos.

We observe breath space when we direct pranic energy, hold or breathe into a specific part of the body. For example in yoga class, it's common for an instructor to encourage breathing into areas that feel tight, compressed, or stuck. As we develop our abilities to feel space in the breath, we can consciously direct the spaciousness to specific areas in our body. We use the spacious quality of our breath to infuse more prana into areas of our body that are experiencing diminished energy flow. Our prana-filled breath opens compressed, weak, or blocked nadi passages so the body can heal, revitalize, and function in its natural state of radiant health.

We explore the space of breath when we observe and control the distance the breath travels into and out of the body. For example, the internal breath may feel shallow and small, traveling only to the upper chest; or the breath may feel rich and full, expanding deep down into the pelvic floor, and even down into the soles of the feet. Pranayama teaches us to experience greater awareness of where the external breath seems to dissolve into the atmosphere beyond our physical body. Just as a drop of water loses its individual nature as it merges and becomes part of a vast ocean, our individual breath is expelled from the body and becomes part of the environmental air we all collectively breathe. This space of our personal external breath is said to extend somewhere from 9 to 12 inches beyond the nostrils before it merges into the surrounding atmosphere. You can feel this for yourself. Simply moisten your palm and place it under your nostrils to feel your breath as you exhale. Slowly move your palm away from your nostrils until you no longer feel your breath. Do this a few times to get a sense of how far your breath extends from your body.

During the kumbhaka phases of pranayama, infinite qualities of space may be profoundly experienced as the breath is suspended either within or outside of the body. As your practice deepens,

you may experience sensations of dissolving the boundaries of
the physical body altogether. You may feel a beautiful experience
of softening and dissolving the space where your skin meets the
surrounding air.

Time and Length of Breath: Matra

Most traditional pranayama techniques call for specific ratios for
inhaling, exhaling, and holds. The breath is counted in time units
called matras (MAH-truh). A matra is approximately one second. Ancient traditions describe measuring the matra by repeating mantras, such as om, or by listening to the beat of your heart.
Listening to meditation music with a steady, rhythmic beat, or
using a metronome or metronome app are effective methods to
time and regulate the matra.

Practicing varying lengths of breath and holds allows us more
mastery over our breath, and can expand and strengthen our
pranic energy. Generally, inhales and retaining the breath
heighten energy. Exhales and holding the breath out release
energy and have a calming effect. We can produce desired results
in our pranic energy by consciously varying the length and ratios
of the four aspects of the breath: inhaling, retaining the breath
in, exhaling, and suspending the breath out. Certain pranayama
techniques apply the bandhas in prescribed times, intensities,
and durations to enhance energetic effects.

As you explore time and length in your pranayama practice, it is
important to understand that longer durations are not necessarily better. You need to focus on quality of breath, state of mind,
and sensations of tension and relaxation. It takes time and prac-

Harmony

Emphasize the inhale to uplift, energize and stimulate. Emphasize the exhale to calm, relax and soothe.

tice to maintain heightened awareness, calmness, and steadiness during conscious breathing techniques; and progress should evolve slowly and incrementally.

Begin your practice with sama vritti, same breath, of equal duration with an easy, comfortable count for inhale and exhale. Practice durations where you feel absolutely no strain or force whatsoever. Keep the same count for inhaling and exhaling. Breathing should feel effortless and smooth. Stay with this duration for a good while and keep with sama vritti.

When moving on, increase the time of breath by only one count, one matra, and stay with that time for a good number of rounds. Many traditional methods of introducing extended breath duration begin by first elongating inhales and exhales. When comfort and mastery of puraka and rechaka are reached then retaining the breath in, antara kumbhaka is added. Bahya kumbhaka is finally introduced only after ease and steadiness are achieved with inhales, exhales and holding the breath in.

It may be tempting to push yourself toward increasingly longer breaths and holds, but it is important to begin with a comfortable, manageable count and stay with it for a good period of time. Don't rush ahead of yourself by extending the breath to a point where you feel strain. Remember that you are building your pranic energies slowly and evenly. Progressing too quickly may over-stimulate the nadi channels, producing erratic pranic energy patterns with undesirable and unhealthy physical, mental and emotional effects. Go for the qualities of steady, slow, smooth, and even. Go for long-term results and not so much for temporary sensations and a sense of rapid achievement. Aim to softly massage your breath and subtle pranas.

Notating the Matra

Matra is commonly notated in the form of a ratio. The inhale is the first number, then duration of holding in, and then the exhale and finally the duration of holding out. For example 1:1:2:1 indicates inhalation, holding in, and holding out are the same length, but the exhalation is twice as long. So if you were following this ratio you may inhale 4, hold in 4, exhale 8 and hold out for 4. Or perhaps inhale 3, hold in 3, exhale 6 and hold out 3. Analyzing the ratio of the pranayama can give you a sense of the desired overall effect of the practice. For example, the 1:1:2:1 pattern would most likely be a relaxing breath because the exhalation is twice as long as the inhalation. Inhales generally energize and exhales generally relax.

Another way pranayama ratios are written notate the duration. A notation for our four-part breath example, sama vritti pranayama, could look like this: 3:3:3:3. Puraka for three beats, antara kumbhaka three beats, rechaka three beats and bahya kumbhaka three beats. A common pranayama ratio for beginners is 4:4:2. Inhale for 4, hold for 4, exhale 2, no hold out.

Counting and Repetition

Some pranayamas are practiced for a particular duration of time and others are practiced for a certain number of repetitions or rounds. It is best to begin your pranayama practice with a small number of repetitions or a short duration. Gradually, over time the number may increase in small increments. A traditional way to count rounds is with the thumb touching the areas between

Time

Some traditions measure lifespan not by the number of years between birth and death, but by the number of breaths between birth and death. Breathe slowly. Live fully.

The Art and Action of Moving Prana

Luminous

Breathe in pure light. Illuminate every atom in your body. Feel the quantum of prana expand exponentially. Radiate joyous luminosity.

the joints of the fingers. I like to start with my thumb at the base of the pinkie finger, successively moving the thumb to each segment my fingers until reaching sthe count of ten.

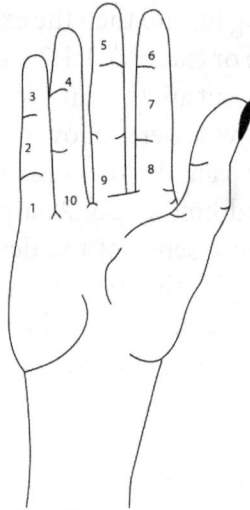

Palm Counting

Mala beads are also used to keep count of the number of repetitions by holding the strand of beads between the fingers and sliding one bead as each round is completed. Malas hold 108 beads, and smaller sizes are made with 27 or 56 beads.

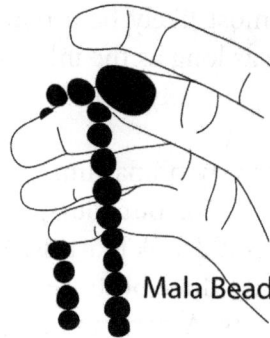

Mala Beads

Four-Part Breath with Bandhas

Now let's enhance our four-part breath example, sama vritti, by adding the bandhas. We will engage mula bandha, uddiyana bandha, and jalandhara bandha during the holds. The bandhas are engaged only during the holding phases, and not during the inhale and exhale. Remember to gently pull up the perineum, draw in the navel, elevate the sternum, and rest the chin into the throat pit. Be mindful and gentle. No forcing or straining. We will use a duration of 3 counts for inhaling, holding in, exhaling, and holding out; 3:3:3:3.

The practice goes like this:

Inhale for 3 counts. Retain the breath and engage root lock, then abdominal lock, then throat lock for 3 counts. Release bandhas. Exhale 3 counts. Suspend the breath out and engage jalandhara bandha, uddiyana, then mula bandha for 3 counts. Release bandhas. Continue to practice three to five rounds, making sure to pause after each round.

Sit quietly and rest for a few moments and notice how you feel. Did the addition of bandhas enhance your practice? Did you feel a heightened experience of pranic energy? Do you perhaps feel a bit more effervescence in your mood and in your body? You should feel energized, fresh, and light throughout your body and mind. If you feel any heaviness or negative effects, avoid engaging the bandhas, and eliminate retention of breath. Continue with a gentle practice, consisting of inhales and exhales, without retentions and bandhas.

Remember to take it very slowly and gently. Practice a few times a day for several minutes. Stay positive and don't get discouraged. Pranayama practices work best with steady and consistent practice. With a slow, mindful, and peaceful approach to your practice, you will be highly rewarded with boundless energy, radiant health, and a strong body and mind.

Suspend

Pause for a brief, infinite moment as your breath transforms from flowing inward into flowing outward. Suspend in space and time as your exhale merges into oneness beyond all form.

The Art and Action of Moving Prana

Essential Pranayamas

*I*nclude the following fundamental breathing techniques in your pranayama practice. Experiment with each technique. You will understand the basic mechanics and general effects right away, but commit to regular daily practice. Consistent practice over time will yield vast benefits and will help you begin to access higher pranas. If you ever feel any type of discomfort, or symptom such as dizziness or nausea, stop the practice and rest. If discomfort persists, do not continue your pranayama practice until you get medical advice regarding your symptoms.

Throat Breath: Ujjayi

In Sanskrit, throat breath is called ujjayi (OO-jay) and means victorious breath. It is important in pranayama, and is the breath used while practicing yoga asanas. In ujjayi, we slightly constrict the glottis to stretch the length of the breath. With the slight constriction of the throat, a soft soothing sound vibration is produced. Ujjayi pranayama has many subtle effects on the body and energy system. The slow, deep breathing immediately calms the mind and body, and the sound of the breath has a peaceful, tranquilizing effect. The vibration of the pharynx directly stimulates the vagus nerve producing a parasympathetic response. This practice is highly effective for insomnia and high blood pressure, and generally all stress-related conditions.

You can practice ujjayi in any position as long as you retain a straight spine. Begin by becoming aware of your natural, spontaneous breath. Breathe smoothly and evenly, and begin to elongate your inhale and exhale. Expand your belly and chest as you inhale. Allow your navel to deflate toward your spine as you breathe out.

Keep your face soft and your shoulders relaxed. Be aware of the area in around the throat pit. Gently part your lips and make a soft, long sound of "haaaaa" as you exhale. Practice a few times. Lengthen your exhale as you make the long sound of "haaaaaaaaaaa" as you exhale.

Next take your palm up to your mouth and exhale into your palm, as if you were fogging up a mirror. Now keep the same breath, but close your lips and remove your palm. As you breathe slowly in and out, you will hear a soft sound like that of gentle ocean waves, or the sound of a baby breathing. Some people compare the sound of ujjayi to that of the Darth Vader character in Star Wars. This is a gentle, soft sound. You should clearly hear it, but not the person on the other side of the room. Feel the subtle vibration at the back of your throat. You should experience a sense of soothing calmness and relaxation.

You may practice ujjayi pranayama for as long as you like. Continue to elongate your inhales and exhales. Keep your pace slow, steady and even. Ujjayi pranayama is much easier to practice than to describe, so jump right in and try it. Relax and experiment with the technique. You will become comfortable with the practice very quickly.

Hear

Listen to the sweetness of your precious breath and infuse divine nectar into each and every thought and each and every word.

Essential Pranayamas

Subtle

Glide your breath gently and slowly along your inner nostril passages, deep into a point between your eyebrows. Smoothly and softly bathe the outer passages of the nostril membranes with your exhale.

Khechari Mudra

You may also practice ujjayi, as well as many other pranayama techniques, with khechari mudra, tongue to upper palate. Khechari mudra (KEH-cha-ree) (MOO-dhruh) helps emphasize the gentle pressure in the throat and enhances the relaxing, soothing effects of ujjayi breathing. The action of the tongue pressing into the upper palate further stimulates the vagus nerve, as it is very close to the surface in this area.

To practice khechari mudra, simply roll your tongue gently up and back and lightly press the underside of the tongue to the upper palate. You may try curling the tongue tip further back, but do not over-stretch the tongue frenulum. You should be comfortable. Hold your tongue in khechari mudra for as long as possible, but do not strain. Whenever you feel uncomfortable, release khechari mudra and let the tongue relax. Come back to the mudra whenever you are ready.

Another, gentler way to practice khechari mudra is to press the tip of the tongue to the upper palate just behind the teeth. Keep the throat, cheeks and face relaxed. As you practice and become more comfortable, try rolling the tongue further back.

Heal

*Master your
breathing and
heal your body,
emotions, mind
and spirit .*

Alternate Nostril Breathing: Nadi Shodhana (Anuloma Viloma)

Alternate nostril breathing is calming, soothing, balancing, and purifying. It is one of the very best practices for calming the mind and relieving stress. Nadi shodhana (NAH-dee) (SHO-dha-nuh) opens and purifies the nadis, the energy pathways that conduct the flow of prana throughout the body. Shodhana means purifica-tion. Nadi shodhana is also called anuloma viloma (ah-noo-LOHM-uh) (vee-LOHM-uh). Anuloma means in the right direction, and viloma means in the opposite direction.

Nadi shodhana is a conscious breathing practice that purifies our pranic energy currents. It operates on all of the internal organs through the autonomic nervous system. Because of its profound physical, emotional, and mental healing benefits, alternate nos-tril breathing is a common pranayama technique used in a wide spectrum of settings. Nadi shodhana is taught in hospitals, clinics, recovery centers, elder care facilities, hospice, corporate offices, schools, spas, fitness centers, and countless other places. This overall feel-good practice reduces cortisol levels, relieves stress and anxiety, balances the nervous system, improves concentra-tion, reduces insomnia and fatigue, reduces blood pressure—the list is seemingly endless! Alternate nostril breathing is very easy to learn and is often the first pranayama method taught to begin-ners. When you practice nadi shodhana your tension melts away and you become peaceful and relaxed. Your nerves are soothed and calmed and you feel and look rested, beautiful and radiant.

Stretch

Inhale and expand yourself very wide. Exhale and stretch yourself long and tall.

The right nostril is the passageway for the pingala nadi. The right channel is active, heating, stimulating, and solar in nature. The left nostril is the passageway for the ida nadi. The left channel is passive, cooling, calming, and lunar in nature. As we practice alternate nostril breathing, we breathe in through one nostril and out the other. By doing so, we purify, balance, and harmonize natural energetic forces within ourselves. Blockages are released, and prana can flow freely, permeating every cell and atom in the body with vital life force energy.

It is important to understand that the nostril linings are a part of the ida and pingala nadi channels. The nostrils play a vital role in efficiently transitioning the breath into and out of the body. Never force breath through the nostrils, or apply strong pressure. The nostrils should be clean, clear, and moist. If you are experiencing a good deal of nasal congestion, wait until the nostrils are clear before practicing alternate nostril breathing.

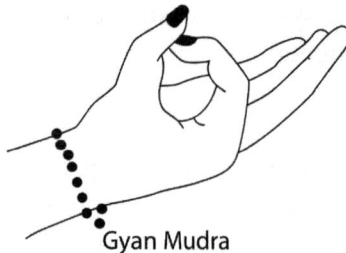

Gyan Mudra

To practice alternate nostril breathing, sit in a comfortable meditative position with the spine straight and tall. Rest the back of the left hand on the left thigh and lightly touch the thumb and first finger together in gyan mudra.

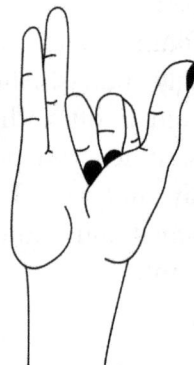

Mrigi Mudra

Make a gentle fist with your right hand, and partially extend your thumb, ring and little fingers.

Exhale all of the breath out through both nostrils, then very lightly touch the pad of the thumb to the right side of your nose, closing the soft flap of skin just below the cartilage. Apply a gentle pressure, only enough to prevent the flow of air in the nostril. Never push the sides of the nostrils in. Be gentle.

Use ujjayi breath as you softly inhale through the left nostril.

Lightly press the pad of your ring finger to close the left nostril. Slowly exhale fully through the right.

Softly inhale through the right nostril. Gently close it with the thumb. Release the left nostril, and softly exhale. This is one round.

Repeat the breath: Inhale left. Close. Exhale right. Inhale right. Close. Exhale left.

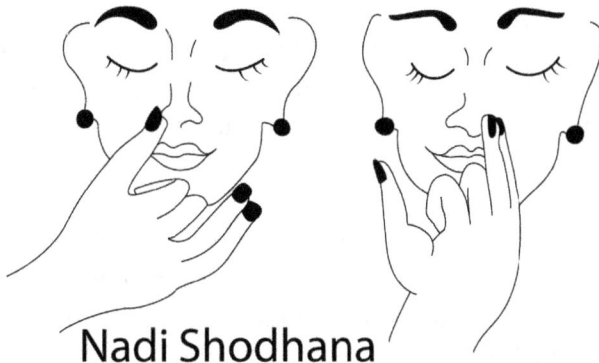

Nadi Shodhana

Continue this breathing pattern for several rounds. Pay attention to the length of the breath as well as the transitions between the inhale and exhale. There should be a smooth, easy transi-

The simple process of shifting awareness from one nostril to the other can lead to profound insights and self-discoveries. The right nostril is associated with concentration, alertness, action. The left nostril is associated with sensitivity, synthesis, calmness.

tion with no pressure, catching or gasping in any way. Adjust the length and pace of your breath until you feel a smooth and easy transition.

Pay attention to how you feel at all times during this practice. You should feel energized, yet balanced, relaxed, and calm. Never force the breath. If you begin to feel uncomfortable in any way, anxious, or light headed, stop the practice and rest.

When you are ready to end the practice, lower the right hand and breathe naturally through both nostrils. Pause and take plenty of time to rest. Observe how you feel.

Right Nostril Breathing: Surya Bhedana

Surya bhedana (SOOR-yuh) (BHEH-duh-nuh) is breathing through the right nostril. It activates the heating, stimulating, and invigorating qualities of the pingala nadi. Surya means sun and bhedana means piercing. Practice right nostril breathing to elevate your energy, improve concentration, and warm the body easily and quickly.

Use ujjayi breath and prepare as you would for alternate nostril breathing. Exhale all of the breath out through both nostrils. Close the left nostril and slowly inhale through the right. Retain the breath in. Gently close the right nostril with the thumb. Release the left nostril, and softly exhale through the left.

Close the left nostril. Softly inhale through the right. Hold the breath in. Lightly close the right nostril and exhale gently through the left.

Continue to inhale through the right and exhale through the left nostril. Close left. Inhale right. Retain breath. Close right. Exhale left. Close left. Inhale right. Retain. Close right. Exhale left.

Continue surya bhedana for several rounds. When you are ready to complete the practice, begin to breathe slowly and evenly through both nostrils. Pause, relax, and notice how you feel. You should feel uplifted and invigorated.

Another variation of surya bhedana is to inhale and exhale exclusively from the right nostril, keeping the left nostril closed the entire time. You may want to practice both versions in separate sessions and compare. Always practice just a little at a time, and keep it gentle. Never overdo it. Using too much pressure or force can disturb the delicate network of nadis and cause undesirable and unhealthy results. Keep your surya bhedana practice energized yet light.

Left Nostril Breathing: Chandra Bhedana

Chandra bhedana (CHAHN-druh) (BHEH-duh-nuh) activates the cooling, soothing qualities of the ida nadi. Chandra means moon and bhedana means piercing. Practice breathing through the left nostril to calm the nervous system, and create a feeling of peace, harmony, and tranquility.

Use gentle ujjayi breath and prepare as you would for alternate nostril breathing. It is also pleasant to practice chandra bhedana while lying down. Exhale all of the breath through both nostrils. Gently close the right nostril and slowly inhale through the left. Gently close the left nostril and softly exhale through the right. Pause with a brief retention of the breath out.

Close the right nostril and softly inhale through the left nostril. Lightly close the left nostril and exhale fully through the right. Gently hold the breath out for just a short pause.

Continue to inhale through the left nostril and exhale through the right. Close right. Inhale left. Close left. Exhale right. Pause. Close right. Inhale left. Close left. Exhale right. Pause.

Continue for a few minutes and notice how you feel. You should feel a nice sense of calm and relaxation.

Another variation of chandra bhedana is to inhale and exhale exclusively from the left nostril, keeping the right nostril closed the entire time. Chandra bhedana is a deeply tranquil and relaxing practice. Enjoy this breath anytime you need to calm down and soothe your nerves.

Shining Skull Breath: Kapalbhati

Kapala is a Sanskrit word meaning skull and bhati means to make clean or to make shine. Kapalbhati (KAH-p-hal-bhah-tee) is a powerful, active, and uplifting pranayama that helps you feel luminous, bright, and alert; making your nostrils, eyes, ears, cheeks, forehead, brain, and entire skull shine! In traditional Hatha yoga, kapalbhati is an essential cleansing and purifying practice, called a shatkarma. Repeated forceful exhalations propel stagnant air from the respiratory system, providing a deep and thorough cleaning.

Kapalbhati cleanses the nasal passages, removes phlegm, and strengthens and tones the circulatory, respiratory, and digestive systems. Kapalbhati purifies and increases energy flow through the nadis. It refreshes and revitalizes the nervous system, relieves stress and depression, improves concentration, strengthens digestion, and reduces anxiety. Regular practice of kapalbhati creates a luminous, radiant glow to your skin.

In Kapalbhati, the exhalation is forceful and active, but the inhale is completely passive. Breath is expelled vigorously from the lungs by pulling in the navel as you exhale. This action pushes the respiratory diaphragm up as the lungs expel air. After the air has been propelled out, the abdomen relaxes, and the breath passively flows in for the inhale.

It is important to master belly breathing before practicing kapalbhati, because this technique requires the navel to draw inward on the exhale. It is a diaphragmatic breath that emphasizes an active exhale and a passive inhale. When you are new to the practice, you may tend to focus too much on the active exhale, but be mindful that the gentle, passive inhale is just as important. It is also important to apply mula bandha (the root lock) during practice to maintain a secure base and to prevent excessive downward pressure, especially on the exhale. Be alert and aware at all times during the practice, and try not to overdo it.

Kapalbhati is a powerful technique. Please consult your physician before practicing this breath technique, especially if you suffer from heart disease, high blood pressure, vertigo, or stroke. Kapalbhati should be practiced on an empty stomach.

Rhythm

Breathe with a steady, rhythmic beat. Pulsate with the natural dance of the universe.

Essential Pranayamas

Experience

Feel the magnificent life force of your prana pulsating through every cell in your body.

Prepare by sitting up straight in a chair, or in your favorite meditation posture. Relax the neck and shoulders, and rest the hands gently on the knees. You may touch the first finger and thumb together in gyan mudra if you like. Keep your entire body relaxed, but upright. Close or soften your eyes. Keep the lips together and teeth slightly apart. Relax your face and your nostrils. Take several slow deep and even breaths.

Begin by expelling all the breath out quickly with vigor, sending your navel back to the spine. Then immediately relax and soften the belly, and allow breath to flow in. This is one round.

Again exhale strongly while contracting the abdominal muscles, propelling the breath quickly out. Then relax the belly as air flows back in. The exhale is strong and powerful, whereas the passive inhale happens effortlessly, naturally, and softly. Inhales will last longer than the powerful exhales. Practice five rounds then rest. Pause, relax, and breathe naturally for a few minutes.

Before beginning another round, practice pulling your navel deeply back to the spine as you exhale. Keep mula bandha engaged as you really pop the navel back to the spine powerfully, forcing the breath to expel out the nose. This is the exhale you want to achieve during kapalbhati. The part of the belly below the navel is the most active part of the exhale and provides a good deal of force to help propel the air up and out. Relax the nostrils, and make sure mula bandha is engaged.

At first you will hear sound in your nostrils as air is forced through them by the powerful exhale. As you become more proficient, try to practice with a subtle constriction of the glottis.

Not quite a ujjayi breath, but just enough to make less sound in the nostrils and a soft sound in the throat. To help achieve this, make sure your inhalations are slow.

When you are ready to begin again, plan to do ten rounds of kapalbhati, maintaining a steady, rhythmic pace. After ten rounds, breathe naturally and notice how you feel. Pause and take plenty of time to rest.

Continue for a few more rounds if you like, making sure you pause and rest in between rounds. A slight euphoric and light-headed feeling is normal. However, if you feel extremely light-headed, dizzy or confused then stop, rest, and quiet the body and mind. When you are ready to begin again, use less force in your exhale. Be aware of all sensations, and allow a feeling of calm energy pulsate through all of the organs of your body and radiate throughout your skin.

Practice kapalbhati comfortably and don't overdo it. Remember, a little goes a long way. Begin slowly with short practice sessions. You may lengthen your practice time by small increments, little by little. It is important to rest after each session.

Take your time. Go at your own pace. If you feel tired or need a break, stop and rest. Be patient, go slowly, and most of all enjoy your pranayama.

Enjoy

Enjoy the power and energy and radiant vitality of your magnificent breath.

. . .

Kapalbhati is a powerful brain tonic and perfect to practice as a pick-me-up for those times when your concentration is foggy, or you feel mentally depleted. Try it for five or six minutes after a stressful day, or during a break from a demanding day at work. Notice your mental clarity and refreshed sense of alertness and attentiveness.

Essential Pranayamas

*Breathe fire,
combustion, the
powerful primal
force of creation.
Ignite your soul.*

Breath of Fire: Bhastrika

Bhastrika (bah-STREE-kah) is a very strong breathing practice similar to kapalbhati, however bhastrika is more powerful and active. Bhastrika means bellows in Sanskrit. Just as a blacksmith uses a bellows to fan the flames with more air to increase heat, bhastrika uses a powerful inhale and exhale to increase heat and energy in the body. While kapalbhati involves an active exhale and passive inhale, breath of fire requires both exhale and inhale to be active.

Bhastrika eliminates toxins and impurities in the physical, emotional, mental, and spiritual layers. It invigorates, revitalizes, and rejuvenates all the systems. Breath of fire is one of the most effective ways to quickly dispel stress, fear, and anxiety while strengthening and stabilizing the nervous system. It reduces inflammation and phlegm, strengthens digestion, purifies and detoxifies the lungs, increases circulation, and improves digestion. Bhastrika expands the flow of prana and recharges the pranic body. It builds stamina, increases mental clarity, and improves focus and concentration. It boosts the immune system, and can help combat cravings and addictions. Bhastrika brings a steady flow of prana to the face and illuminates the skin with a radiant, clear, and healthy glow.

It is important to master belly breathing before practicing breath of fire, because this technique requires the navel to draw inward on the exhale and expand outward on the inhale. Bhastrika must be practiced on an empty stomach. It is also important to apply mula bandha (the root lock) throughout the practice to maintain a secure base and to prevent excess downward pressure. Maintain heightened, conscious awareness of your breath at all times while practicing bhastrika.

· · ·

Bhastrika is a strong, energizing practice. Consult your physician before practicing this breath technique if you suffer from: heart disease, high blood pressure, vertigo, or stroke. Be aware of how you feel at all times during this practice. Keep your practice sessions short, a little goes a long way.

Let's begin by sitting up straight in a chair, or in your favorite meditation posture. Relax the neck and shoulders and rest your hands gently on your knees. Touch the first fingers and thumbs together in gyan mudra if you like. Keep the entire body relaxed and upright with a straight spine. Close your eyes. Keep the lips together and teeth slightly apart. Breathe in deeply and slowly, and exhale smoothly and completely. Relax and begin belly breathing.

Slightly lift mula bandha and feel the navel press back toward the spine as you exhale. Now begin to breathe in and out quickly and forcefully through the nostrils, pulsing the navel in a steady rhythm. The front, back, and sides of chest will move somewhat in this practice, but the focus is on the abdominal area. The abdomen pumps in and out with longer duration of the inhale than exhale. Breath is steady and rapid. The belly quickly relaxes on each inhale and rapidly forces the breath out on the exhale. Try to keep a steady, even beat while you breathe in and out vigorously with the navel pumping. Continue for thirty seconds.

To stop the practice, take in a deep, slow inhale. Apply mula bandha, uddiyana bandha, jalandhara bandha, and retain the breath in. Gently release the bandhas and exhale slowly. Relax, breathe slowly, deeply and evenly, and notice how you feel.

Exhilarate

Pranayama evokes amazing, exciting, awesome energy!

Repeat for another cycle if desired. This time extend your practice to one minute, then rest.

It's normal to feel a little light headed and slightly dizzy at first. But if you feel extremely dizzy, or disoriented, stop, relax, and quiet the body and mind for a good period of time. When you have rested and begin another session, use less force and practice for a shorter duration.

It's important to keep a steady rhythm. Keep a manageable pace, with an even volume of air that comes in and out. As you become proficient, your pace will increase, but don't let the volume of air diminish. If you find that speeding up your rhythm decreases the volume of air coming in and out, slow down and concentrate more. Soften your face, relax your shoulders down, and be aware of the nostril linings and openings.

Practice bhastrika comfortably on your own, but don't overdo it. Begin very slowly with short practice sessions. You may lengthen your practice time by very small increments, little by little. Take plenty of time to rest after each session.

Remember, it takes time and lots of practice to develop mastery over the breath of fire. Be patient, be gentle, enjoy the pranayama, and learn to experience subtle effects over time.

• • •

Bhastrika is one of the most powerful pranayama practices. It is important to practice with keen awareness and steadiness. Bhastrika brings together prana and apana at the navel center, creating ideal pranic conditions for kundalini energy to activate and arise up through the sushumna. Be aware during the finishing kumbhaka phase, and energetically pull prana up from the base of the body.

Breath of Fire: Ego Eradicator

A staple in the practice of kundalini yoga as taught by Yogi Bhajan, is a pranayama called ego eradicator that combines an extended arm position with breath of fire. Yogi Bhajan taught breath of fire in a fun, colorful way. He instructed beginners to first stick out the tongue and imagine panting through your mouth like a dog. Feel the navel pulse in and out with each breath. Breathe rapidly. Establish a steady rhythm, then close your mouth so you are breathing at the same speed, but only through your nose.

To practice the powerful ego eradicator pranayama, sit up tall and straight. Extend your arms overhead and uplift them out to the sides at a sixty-degree angle. This is approximately at the ten o'clock and two o'clock position. Keep your arms taught and strong with elbows straight. Extend your thumbs away from the hands, and stretch your fingers and palms. Then curl your fingers so that the fingertips press into the mounds at the base of each finger. Keep the thumbs up and out like a hitchhiker. Keep your shoulders and neck relaxed while the arms are strong, straight, and powerful.

Keep the arms extended in this position and begin breath of fire. Imagine that your thumbs are like cosmic antennae pulling prana into your body. The navel forcefully pulses inward on every exhale. Increase the pace to two exhales per second. Practice ego eradicator for one to three minutes.

Join

Join in. We're all breathing the same air, sharing a common prana. Our beautiful breath is keeping us all alive!

Revitalize

Feel your thoughts, speech, and actions joyfully dance to the delightful rhythm of your breath.

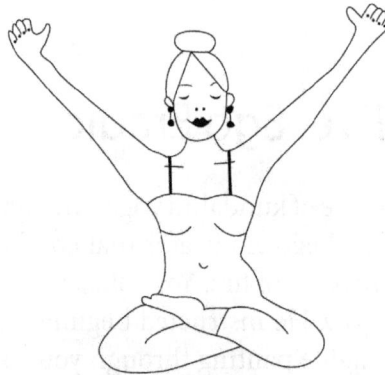

Ego Eradicator

To end the practice, take a long, deep inhale as you raise your arms up straight overhead. Touch the tips of your thumbs together, open your fingers, and hold your breath for as long as you feel comfortable.

When you are ready to exhale, sweep your arms out and down, and very slowly let the breath release out through your nose as you slowly lower your arms. Touch your fingertips to the surface beneath you to ground your energy down. As the arms sweep down, imagine you charging your pranic field around your body.

Sit still for several minutes, relax, and observe how you feel.

Interrupted Breath: Viloma

Viloma (vee-LOH-muh) teaches you to lengthen the breath and to gain mastery and control of the diaphragm. Viloma means against the flow, or against the grain, and literally against the hair. Vi means against, and loma means hair. When we practice viloma, we breathe against the grain, or interrupt the natural flow of our breath. We segment the inhales and exhales with brief, rhythmic pauses in the breath flow. By interrupting the natural flow, it takes longer to complete a full breath cycle.

Segmenting the breath builds strength and flexibility in the diaphragm, and increases stamina and concentration. Viloma is an effective pranayama to help restore vitality when recovering from an illness or from fatigue. It is soothing, elevates mood, encourages positivity and is stabilizing and strengthening.

When learning viloma, it may be helpful to practice while lying on your back so that you can feel stable, secure, and can feel the full circumference of the respiratory diaphragm. It is relaxing and grounding to feel your back fully supported. You should master belly breathing before trying viloma, and it is helpful to know ujjayi breath. Until you are familiar with the technique, it is a common tendency to tighten the belly and expand the chest, as in reverse breathing. It's important to keep the chest, neck, and shoulders completely relaxed, and use the navel and diaphragm to pause the breath. Don't constrict the chest.

Begin by lying down on your back. Your knees may be bent and the soles of your feet pressing into the surface below, so you can feel the entire surface of the back body. Close your eyes and breathe slowly, deeply, and evenly. Begin slow belly breathing with a very gentle ujjayi. As your breath becomes smooth and rhythmic, you may elongate your legs, but try not to arch the lower back.

To begin viloma pranayama, start to breathe in for a couple of seconds then pause. Bring in a bit more breath, and pause. Breathe in a little, pause. Breathe in a little, pause. Finally fill the lungs to capacity without straining. Very slowly and steadily exhale.

Essential Pranayamas

Silky

Slowly and gently inhale through the very center of the nostrils, without making the slightest disturbance in the nasal lining. Smoothly transition to exhale through the center of the nostrils, without causing a flutter of the fine hairs lining the nostril passages.

Try it again. Without straining, inhale in several segments, pausing and stabilizing at each stop. You do not release the diaphragm at the pauses. Gently still the diaphragm without tightly gripping it. Hold in briefly at the very top when the lungs are fully inflated if you like. Slowly and evenly breathe out.

Continue practicing viloma pranayama for as long as you are comfortable. To end the practice, breathe spontaneously and naturally. Take plenty of time to rest and notice how you feel.

It may help to imagine the breath as a stream of fluid, slowly flowing into the body as if it is being poured from a pitcher. The breath flows in, stops, flows in a little more, stops, flows a little more, and stops, until the body is full. Try to keep relaxed and in control of the flow and stops. If you begin to feel anxious or experience any straining, simply take fewer stops of shorter duration.

Viloma is also practiced on the exhalation. Practice just as you would on the inhale, but instead take an interrupted exhalation and long smooth inhale. Become familiar with both, and notice the differences in the way you feel with each technique.

Humming Bee Breath: Bhramari

Bhramari (BHRAH-mah-ree) means bee in Sanskrit. When practicing bhramari you make a soft humming sound as you breathe out, resembling the sound made by a bee. Bhramari breath is deeply soothing and relaxing. The soft sound and gentle vibrations stimulate the parasympathetic nervous system to balance and harmonize the body and emotions. The light pressure of closing the ear flaps further stimulates the vagus nerve in the ear canal, enhancing the parasympathetic response. Bhramari reduces blood pressure, helps prevent insomnia, and alleviates tension, anxiety, and overall stress. The soothing effects help foster a pleasant, positive attitude to life's challenges.

Begin by sitting in any comfortable posture. Slowly breathe deeply and evenly, and prepare to fully relax. Close your eyes, keep the lips together and teeth slightly parted.

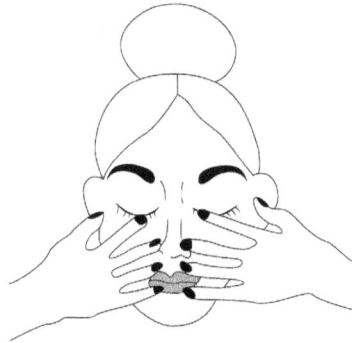

Bhramari

Now gently close the flaps of your ears very lightly with your thumbs. Softly place your index and middle fingertips on the closed eyes, without placing any pressure on the eyeball. Your ring and pinkie fingers will rest on your cheeks.

Inhale softly. While gently exhaling, make a soft humming sound and feel the subtle vibrations of the humming inside your head. Hum for the entire duration of the exhale.

Continue to inhale gently and hum softly as you slowly exhale. Practice bhramari for as long as you like. Then keep your eyes closed, lower your hands, and sit in silence. Observe how you feel.

Regular pranayama practice brings about laser-beam focus and concentration. The yogis call this ekagrata – one pointed focus.

The breath is the meeting place of body, mind and spirit.

Cooling Breath: Sitali

Sitali pranayama (SEE-tah-lee) cools, soothes and relaxes the system. It quenches thirst and reduces hunger. Sitali practice eases fever and can alleviate indigestion. Try sitali any time you feel overheated and need to cool down.

Sitali may be practiced in any comfortable posture. Begin by opening the mouth then purse your lips into an 'O' shape. Curl your tongue into a 'U' shape, protrude your tongue out slightly beyond your lips, and draw air in through the tongue as if you were sipping through a straw. Make your inhale slow and deep. Close your lips and exhale slowly through your nostrils.

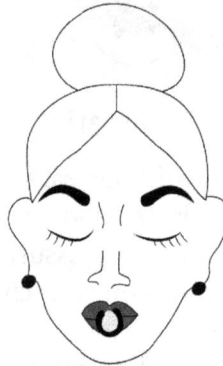

Sitali

Continue to inhale slowly through the curled tongue, close the mouth, and exhale through the nose. Practice for as long as you like then rest. Notice if you feel refreshed, awake and cool.

Refreshing Breath: Sitkari

You may also want to practice a similar breath called Sitkari (SEET-kah-ree), hissing breath. The process is very similar to sitali, however the breath comes in around the sides of the teeth instead of through the curled tongue.

To practice sitkari, separate the teeth ever so slightly, widen the sides of the mouth, and place the tip the tongue just behind front teeth and touching the upper palate. Sip in the air so it swirls in along the sides of the teeth and inner cheek lining, making a hissing sound. Then close the lips, relax the tongue, and exhale through the nose.

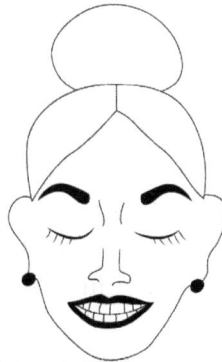

Seetkari

Practice sitkari for several minutes then rest. You should feel refreshed, calm, cool, and awake.

Lion Breath: Simhasana

Simha means lion and asana means seat or pose. Simhasana (sim-HA-sah-nuh) is a powerful cleansing breath. It purifies and detoxifies the system and strengthens the thyroid. It relaxes and tones the facial muscles, and produces a pleasant, positive feeling. It builds confidence and reduces feelings of anxiety and fear.

Lion breath may be practiced in any posture, but is commonly practiced in a kneeling position with the buttocks resting on the backs of your heels. The palms are pressing into the thighs or knees with the arms strong and elongated. You may also lean forward slightly and press your palms down into the floor, with the fingers pointing back toward the body, and inner wrists and elbows facing forward.

Breathe in fully and deeply through your nose. Open your mouth, widen, and stick out your tongue, as if you are reaching the tongue tip down to your chin. You will look like a mighty lion preparing to roar. As you exhale, pull your eyeballs up and in toward the center of your eyebrows in shambhavi mudra and exhale powerfully making a deep "haaaaaaa" sound, like a roar.

Close your mouth, soften the eyes, and inhale from your nose. Exhale again powerfully, sticking out the tongue and making it wide, with a deep roar of "haaaaaaaa."

Practice several times. When you are ready to end the practice, come to a comfortable resting posture, relax, and notice how you feel.

Shambhavi Mudra: Eyebrow Center Gazing

Concentrate

Send breath like a laser beam deep into a single point.

Simhasana, as well as many other pranayama techniques are enhanced with shambhavi mudra (sham-BHAH-vhee) (MOO-dhruh), eyebrow center gazing. The eyeballs roll up and in as if gazing inside the skull just behind the center of the eyebrows. The eyes should remain closed, although it is possible to practice shambhavi mudra with the eyes open. It is important to be gentle and never strain when practicing this mudra.

Shambhavi mudra applies gentle pressure on the optical nerve. This action stimulates the vagus nerve and produces a parasympathetic, relaxing response. The pineal gland is stimulated as conscious awareness and pranic flow is directed into ajna chakra, the eyebrow center. By applying mula bandha and shambhavi mudra simultaneously, pranic flow from the base to the upper centers is enhanced. Try shambhavi mudra with mula bandha and antara kumbhaka. Be very gentle as the nerves in the eyes and inner head area are very delicate.

Shambhavi mudra activates the pineal gland and soothes the nerves. With practice, concentration and mental stability are increased, and a calm sense of inner tranquility develops. You will find that you naturally ease into a state of peaceful meditation following this practice.

Practices and Sequences

You now have all of the building blocks to put together a personal practice for yourself. Establish a regular pranayama habit. The techniques you select may vary, but practice every day, several times a day, with the goal of breathing consciously and mindfully in each and every breath of your life.

– Practices –

Invocation of Energy, Prana Mudra

This beautiful practice is the best way to begin each day. As we practice prana mudra, we use our breath, retentions, conscious awareness, and mudras to bring vital prana up and throughout the body. This awakens the powerful prana shakti, universal energy, and circulates it throughout the body. We feel the prana rise up in one full inhalation from the root chakra to the navel, to the heart center, to the throat center, and throughout the centers in the head. We keep awareness of our prana as it descends back down to muladhara chakra on the exhale.

Prana mudra is ideally done at sunrise, but may be practiced any time you would like an overall lift and expansion of your energetic body. Prana mudra pulls up prana that is lying stagnant and dormant in the lower parts of the body, bringing it upward through the nadis to the highest crown of the head. Vital prana is distributed throughout the entire body and infused into all of the bodily systems. Prana mudra builds vitality and fosters a confident, optimistic attitude for all of your endeavors. This practice bathes the subtle energy channels with pure life force energy and builds pranic awareness of the nadis and chakra energy centers. Regular practice of prana mudra increases your ability to feel subtle pranas and to consciously direct prana into specific areas of your body. It builds stamina and allows you to develop progressively longer breaths and retentions.

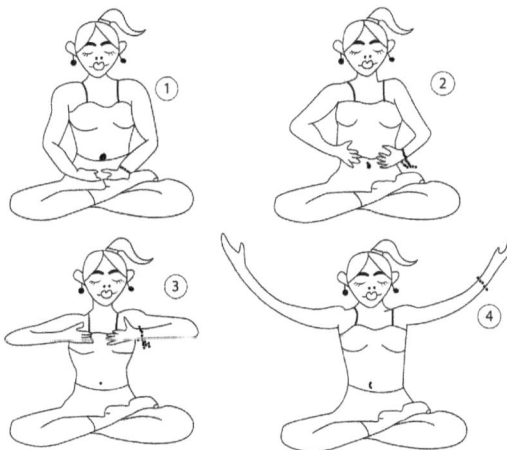

Prana Mudra

To begin, sit in a comfortable posture with the spine straight and tall. With the palms facing up, place your left hand in your right and rest both hands on your lap in bhairava mudra (by-RHAH-vuh) (MOO-dhruh). Close your eyes and relax the entire body. Breathe slowly, deeply and evenly for a few moments until you feel settled.

Abundance

Very, very long inhale. Exhale all at once.

Take in a deep inhale then exhale every ounce of breath out of the body, pulling in the abdomen and uddiyana bandha to help expel all of the breath. Keep the breath held out and apply mula bandha. Keep bahya kumbhaka for as long as comfortably possible while focusing on the root chakra.

Release mula bandha as you begin to slowly inhale. Soften the belly and bring in as much breath into the abdomen as you can, while raising your hands up in front of your navel. Your body, arms, and hands stay completely relaxed. Keep the fingers apart, palms facing the body, and hold the hands close to one another, but not touching. Feel yourself pulling prana up from muladhara chakra to the navel center, synchronizing the movement of your hands rising up with your inhalation.

Keep inhaling and pull the prana up into anahata chakra, while raising the hands up in front of your heart center. Expand your ribcage and chest, and feel pranic energy flow up from manipura chakra to anahata.

Stay relaxed as you continue inhaling up into the clavicles, shoulders, and throat while bringing your hands in front of the throat pit. Feel vital energy flood upwards from the heart center to vishuddhi chakra.

Retain your breath as you extend your arms out to your sides, palms up at the level of your ears. Concentrate on feeling your prana bathe ajna chakra between your eyebrows, bindu (BIN-doo) at the back of the skull, and sahasrara chakra at the crown of your head. Keep antara kumbhaka for as long as possible, feeling prana vibrate through every cell and atom of your body and radiate through every pore of your skin. Stay vibrant and relaxed. Do not strain.

Slowly exhale with concentrated awareness, reversing your hand movements, while taking the prana downwards through the throat, heart, navel, and root chakras. Apply mula bandha and concentrate on muladhara chakra as prana reaches the base at the end of the exhalation.

Repeat for several rounds. You may want to take a deep, full breath between rounds. When you are ready to complete your practice, relax and breathe naturally and slowly. Notice your subtle energies, and observe how you feel.

To enhance your prana mudra practice, add awareness of the pancha vayus. The breath and arm movements remain the same, and you add your conscious awareness of pranic sensations of the pancha vayus. To begin, feel the downward moving, heavier qualities of apana vayu below the navel to the perineum. As you bring awareness up to the navel, be aware of the circular, assimilating energy of samana vayu. When your awareness arises to the heart center, feel the expansive and inspiring sensations of prana vayu. As you bring awareness to the throat center, be aware of uplifting, ascending energy of udana vayu in the head. As you retain your breath and spread your arms, feel your entire body supported by the radiant prana of vyana vayu. Feel your entire body filled and surrounded by vibrant, sparkling prana. Reverse the process as you exhale down to the root.

Relaxing Breath 4:7:8

This practice comes from Dr. Andrew Weil. He recommends this practice to his patients for reducing stress and anxiety, and for building stability and confidence. It is helpful to practice the relaxing breath 4:7:8 pattern with the help of a metronome, or

Breathe in deep every possibility, breathe out and release every tie that binds you.

metronome app, to keep a steady count. It is also a nice preparation to practice bhastrika for one minute to energize and warm up.

Begin by sitting comfortably and place the tip of your tongue lightly against the upper palate behind the front teeth. Keep the lips together, teeth slightly apart.

Begin the breathing pattern. Exhale all breath out then take a long inhale quietly through the nose for the count of four. Hold the breath in for the count of seven. Exhale all the breath out through mouth noisily around the tongue, making a whooshing sound for the count of eight. This is one round.

Inhale through the nostrils for the count of four. Hold for the count of seven. Exhale through the mouth for the count of eight.

Repeat a total of four rounds, several times daily.

Two Beat Viloma

This viloma practice is an excellent way to increase breath control and stamina, and is a fabulous way to practice fluid breath retentions. You will need to maintain a steady beat, so using a metronome or metronome app is helpful here. You may also use the steady rhythm of your heartbeat to keep the matra for this practice.

This pranayama may be practiced in any comfortable position. Make sure to stay relaxed and keep your spine straight. Remember that concentration on your breath and establishing a steady beat is the objective. It is not important to increase the lung volume or length of retentions. Try not to feel that you must achieve—simply create awareness, steadiness, and rhythm. Stay relaxed the entire time. If retentions begin to cause tightness or stiffness, then you are trying too hard. Begin breathing slowly, deeply and evenly. Establish a steady matra either with a metronome or with your heartbeat.

The first phase is viloma during the inhalation. Breathe in for two beats. Pause the breath for two beats. Breathe in for two more beats then suspend the breath for two beats. Breathe in for two, pause for two, until the lungs are nearly full. Now take in a deep, full, yogic, three part breath, filling up the lower belly, chest, and upper clavicle area. Hold the breath in for as long as you can without straining, then slowly exhale all of the breath out.

Without pausing, start the round again. Breathe in for two beats and suspend for two beats, over and over until lungs are full. Take in a big, deep breath then hold the breath in. Without straining or gasping, slowly and smoothly exhale all of the breath out of the lungs. Repeat this cycle five times.

The next phase is viloma on the exhalation. Slowly inhale deeply filling up the lower belly, chest and upper clavicle area. Exhale for two beats, suspend the breath for two beats. Exhale for two more beats then hold the breath for two beats. Continue this pattern until all the breath is out, then hold the breath out for as long as comfortable.

Right away take in a deep, yogic breath. Exhale two beats, hold two, exhale two, suspend two, exhale two, hold two until all the breath is out. Hold the breath out. Repeat this cycle five times.

*Make your
breath so pure
and light that it
feels as though
you are not
breathing at all.*

After five cycles of two beat viloma inhaling, and five cycles of two beat viloma exhaling, take a long rest. It's best to lie down and breathe normally, allowing the benefits of your pranayama to permeate through your body, mind, emotions, and spirit.

At first, you will take only a few inhales and pauses to fill the lungs, and just a few exhales and pauses to empty the lungs. But with practice, over time you will be able to take more inhale/pauses and exhale/pauses because your breath control and stamina will improve. Remember, the count always remains at two. You progress by increasing the number of breath/pause steps it takes to either fill or empty the lungs.

Expansive Breath Retention

This practice evokes an uplifting, expansive feeling while retaining the breath in. It allows you to view life's circumstances from an elevated vantage point. It helps you overcome feelings of insecurity and fear. Expanding your awareness with breath retention helps you achieve positive breakthroughs, overcome challenging obstacles, and deal with negative life patterns.

You will breathe in, hold while imagining the body inflating larger-than-life size, and then exhale fully. There are no specific counts or matras for this breath. It requires you to pay very keen attention to sensations in the body and mind to determine the durations of your inhale and retention. You should remain calm and relaxed through the practice. No straining or forcing in any way. It is best to approach this practice with the intent to stay just below your capacity. So if you feel you can retain the breath

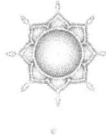

for ten counts, then only retain for eight or seven. Less is more. Expansive breath retention may be practiced in a seated posture or lying down.

Start by coming to a comfortable seated or reclining posture with the spine straight. Relax and breathe slowly and deeply for a few moments.

To begin, exhale all of the breath out of the body. Inhale slowly and deeply into the belly, hold your breath in for as long as comfortable—don't force it. Imagine your whole body growing larger and larger and larger. Inflate and expand your body as big as you can imagine. Then without gasping or straining, exhale fully. Relax and take a normal, deep breath.

Repeat up to five times. Then completely rest, be still, and notice your feelings and insights.

Remember, a little goes a long way. Use caution and sound judgment when holding your breath, never force or strain. Always consult a physician if you have a condition that would make it inadvisable to practice breath retention.

Confidence Boosting Breath

In this breath, we powerfully propel the breath out of the body through pursed lips. If you like to use guided imagery, you may want to imagine blowing away your concern, issue, problem, or troublesome situation far out of your body and mind. Use this strong exhaling practice to breathe away your worries.

Grace

When you are upset and feeling bad, just take a long deep breath.

Close your lips and draw in a slow, deep breath through your nostrils. Relax your chest and shoulders expand your lungs as much as you can, especially at the very top. Stay relaxed and pause briefly. Softly purse your lips so they form a round "o" shape without puffing out the cheeks. Quickly expel every ounce of your breath out through the pursed lips.

Repeat several times. Stop, rest, and be aware of how you feel.

Conscious Exhale Counting

This practice is very simple, however, it requires tremendous concentration. You will focus your mind intently to count the duration of your exhales. Conscious exhale counting breath evokes a deeply relaxing, pleasant meditative state, and improves memory and concentration. It is also a soothing way to relax in bed before falling asleep.

Sit in a comfortable position, or lie down on your back. Close your eyes and breathe slowly, deeply and naturally for a few minutes.

To begin the practice, count "one" to yourself as you exhale.

The next time you exhale, mentally count "two," and so on until you get to "five."

Once you reach "five", begin a new cycle, silently counting "one" on the next exhalation.

Never count higher than "five," on the exhale. If you find yourself counting higher, simply begin again at "one." Focus and discipline your mind.

Repeat for as many cycles as you like. Practice regularly and consistently, and try to increase the number of rounds each time you practice.

Gradual Lengthening Breath

This practice helps you build strength, stamina, and increased concentration by steadily increasing the length of the inhale, retention, and exhalation. This is a sama vritti pranayama practice with the inhale, exhale, and retentions of equal duration. It is important to be gentle with yourself. Never force or strain. Your breath will lengthen naturally and gradually with regular consistent practice. Don't go beyond your capacity. There should never be any gasping or straining. It may also be helpful to practice with the steady rhythm of a metronome or metronome app.

Practice in any comfortable posture. Relax and take several deep, slow and even breaths. Exhale all the breath out.

Using ujjayi breath, begin by slowly inhaling to the count of four. Hold for four counts. Exhale four counts. This is one round. Breathe 4:4:4 for several rounds.

If you are ready to lengthen the breath, add one count. 5:5:5. Breathe 5:5:5 for several rounds. Be comfortable and relaxed. The breath should flow effortlessly.

Ask

Inhale slowly and deeply and ask for your heart's desire. Let this request come from the purist, truest, deepest source of your breath. Feel into this place. Suspend. Release your breath and release the desire. Fully let it go.

If you are ready to end the practice, stop and rest. If you would like to continue, add one count to breathe 6:6:6. Stay with the count for a good while before adding on for 7:7:7.

Continue adding one count, making sure you remain fully relaxed with no strain. Stay at a count just below your capacity. Instead of pushing yourself to reach a higher count, focus on deepening and refining your awareness with ease and comfort to experience a richer, fuller understanding of your pranic energies.

When you are ready to end the practice, breathe naturally and take plenty of time to pause and rest. Notice how you feel.

Practice regularly. Make a goal to practice twice a day for a week and stick to it. Notice the positive changes in your life!

Tibetan 9 Round Breath: Gentle Version

This classic breath pattern involves alternate nostril breathing—slowly and gently. It is a balancing, soothing, and restorative pattern. Sages claim this breath dissolves attachments, desire, anger, hatred, ignorance, and confusion. Ancient versions of this breath practice incorporate visualizing prana traveling through the ida, pingala, and sushumna nadi channels as colored smoke. Red light is visualized as breath is inhaled through the right channel, pingala. White light is visualized as breath is inhaled through the left channel, or ida. Exhales are visualized with black smoke carrying away toxins, impurities, and residues from the body.

This version of Tibetan nine breaths can be practiced in any comfortable posture. Relax and breathe gently and naturally. The right hand thumb and ring fingers are used to close the nostrils, and the left hand rests softly down. You may place the left thumb and index finger together in gyan mudra if you like.

Begin by exhaling all of the breath out. Use your right thumb to gently close the right nostril. Slowly breathe in through the left nostril, feeling the breath travel through ida nadi down into the base of the body. Close the left nostril with the right ring finger and softly, and slowly exhale through the right nostril. Feel the breath rise up through the right passage, pingala nadi, and out the right nostril. Repeat this three times.

Next, reverse the pattern. Gently breathe in through the right nostril and out through the left for three repetitions, visualizing the prana travel through the nadis.

Finally, lower your hand and very slowly and softly breathe in and out of both nostrils evenly three times. Imagine the breath traveling through the spinal passage, sushumna nadi.

Pause and rest. Sit silently with your eyes closed for a good while. Notice how you feel.

You may repeat for several rounds if you like. Be certain to rest and sit silently after each session.

Comfort

Breathe in tenderly, gently, easily. Receive the soft, gentle, loving inner caress of your sweet breath. Softly float your precious breath away to merge into the vast space beyond. Soothe your soul.

Celebrate

Joyfully celebrate your breath. Celebrate each and every life-sustaining breath. Celebrate the ups, celebrate the downs, and rejoice in the infinite, blissful space between.

Tibetan 9 Round Breath: Active Version

This classic breath pattern involves alternate nostril breathing with breath retention and active exhalations. It is powerful, invigorating, strengthening, and heightens awareness.

The breath is exhaled quickly in this practice; however, it is very important make sure to maintain heightened awareness and control of the outbreath, so that very little pressure is exerted against the nasal walls. Do this by applying mula bandha and uddiyana bandha as you expel the breath. The nostril linings should stay relatively undisturbed, with the breath flowing smoothly through the center of the nostrils. You may also add nadi color visualizations, as described in the gentle version of Tibetan 9 Round Breath.

Practice this active version of Tibetan 9 Round Breath in a comfortable, seated posture with the spine very straight. Breathe fully, gently, and naturally. The right hand thumb and ring fingers are used to close the nostrils, and the left hand rests softly down. You may place the left thumb and index finger together in gyan mudra if you like.

Begin by exhaling all the breath out. Gently close the right nostril with your right thumb. Slowly breathe in through the left nostril. Feel the lungs slowly fill. Create an exaggerated slow deep fill, as if you are breathing in slow motion. Retain the breath for as long as is comfortable. Close the left nostril, and exhale all at once out the right nostril pulling in mula bandha and uddiyana bandha. Do this three times.

Next reverse the pattern. Slowly breathe in through the right nostril, filling the lungs fully. Hold the breath in. Then quickly exhale out the left nostril, engaging the root and abdominal locks. Do this three times.

Finally, take a slow fill of the lungs to capacity, as you slowly draw breath in through both nostrils. Hold the breath for as long as you can comfortably without strain. Then quickly exhale all at once through both nostrils.

Pause, rest, and sit silently in mindful meditation.

Proceed

Proceed through life with only the highest most divine pranas in everything you do.

Walking Pranayama

When you practice pranayama consistently, you begin to develop continued, sustained awareness of your breath. Observing your breath becomes effortless. Your mind becomes centered and calm. Your concentration improves. You handle life's ups and downs with grace and ease. Stress seems to melt away. Your skin becomes luminous. You feel healthy, happy, and youthful. But most of us have very busy days, and it can sometimes present a challenge to pause for a sitting pranayama practice. Many pranayamas can be practiced anytime, anywhere. Practicing conscious breathing while walking is a great way to work pranayama into a busy day.

The easiest form of walking pranayama is timing your breath with your steps. Simply find a rhythm. There is no right or wrong way to do this. Perhaps you take five steps per inhale and five

When you
release your
breath out of
your body, it
has no end. It
travels past the
boundaries of
our solar system,
our galaxy, our
universe and
beyond, merging
with infinite
divine source.
As you receive a
new breath into
the body, the
entire cosmos is
breathing you.

steps per exhale. Or walk very briskly, taking ten steps per inhale and ten steps per exhale. Maybe you take fifteen steps on the inhale, then exhale all at once. The possibilities are endless.

The revered Swami Sivananda Saraswati describes a walking pranayama timing the breath and steps to the chant of om. He gives the duration as 3:12:6. Inhale three, hold twelve, and exhale six. As you are walking, inhale slowly for three steps, silently chanting om with each step. Retain the breath for twelve steps, silently chanting om on each step. Exhale slowly for six om steps. Then breathe naturally for twelve steps, still mentally chanting om with each step. Repeat for as many cycles as you like.

Swami Sivananda also mentions that kapalbhati is an invigorating pranayama that pairs well with walking. Simply walk briskly, using vigorous kapalbhati breathing. Make sure to keep mula bandha engaged and emphasize navel pumps on the exhale.

Heartbeat Rhythm Breathing

Heartbeat rhythm breathing is both a pranayama and a meditation that gently tunes you in to the rhythm of your heart. It is soothing, comforting, quieting, balancing, and easy to master. By synchronizing your breathing with the beat of your heart, all the while maintaining focus, conscious awareness of these organic rhythms, you are nurtured into a deep meditative state. The body and mind layers are comforted by allowing the supportive pulse of internal pranas be heard, felt, and profoundly experienced. Life can seem overwhelming when we are presented with external chaos, difficulties, problems, powerful emotions, challenges, and traumas. We become imbalanced and out of synch when we align ourselves disproportionately to external forces. Our natural, healthy internal rhythms help us maintain a smooth, regular flow of prana throughout our physical, mental, emotional, intellectual, and spiritual layers. Our naturally pulsating rhythms keep our internal systems functioning in harmony, and keep us in sync with the larger organic rhythms of our human communities, nature, our planet, and the vast cosmos.

Heartbeat rhythm breathing is a beautiful practice to soothe and comfort yourself when life just seems too much, and you are having trouble coping. It can be particularly effective when going through times of grief, loss, heartbreak, sadness, or loneliness.

You can practice heartbeat rhythm breathing in any posture, but keep in mind that you will need to take your own pulse for an extended period of time. There are several areas in the body to feel your pulse. You may want to experiment and try heartbeat rhythm breathing while feeling your pulse in the wrist, chest, abdomen, or neck. However, for this practice, it best to feel the pulse in your wrist so that the movements of the chest and abdomen do not interfere with your focused awareness on the heartbeat.

To find the pulse in your wrist, gently press the tips of your first two or three fingers to your inner wrist until you feel your pulse. Make sure you use a very light touch, just enough to feel your heartbeat.

Find a comfortable position either seated or lying down and make the spine straight. Relax your neck and shoulders. Close your eyes and begin to breathe slowly, deeply, and evenly.

Practices and Sequences

Shine

Feel your breath shine like the sun.

Rest your arms in your lap or on your body to begin finding your pulse. Once you find it, simply relax and feel the beat. Stay with this for a few moments. You do not need to anything but simply feel the pulse of your heart.

Begin to become aware of your breathing. Breathe slowly and effortlessly. Maintain awareness of your heartbeat. Simultaneously expand your focused attention to the beat of your heart and your breathing.

Now inhale for four heartbeats and exhale for four heartbeats. Breathe like this for a while. Inhale and exhale for four heartbeats, sama vritti.

After a while, extend your inhale and exhale to last for five heartbeats. Stay with this duration for a few minutes.

Extend your inhale and exhale to six heartbeats. Breathe in this rhythm for a while. Continue to lengthen your duration by one count in this way, always maintaining a smooth transition between breaths. If the breath catches, or becomes choppy in between, shorten the duration until your breath flows smoothly and evenly.

When you are ready to end the practice, breathe naturally and spontaneously. Pause, rest, and notice how you feel. Sit quietly in mindful meditation for a while.

Sparkling Energy Breath

This practice involves interrupted breathing, viloma. Sparkling energy breath is an uplifting, energizing pranayama and is an excellent way to bring an exciting, effervescent quality into your day. Sparkling energy breath is good for dealing with confusion, depression, and anxiety. It clears the mind and brings about a positive outlook.

Practice sparkling energy breath in a comfortable seated position with the spine straight and tall. Relax the shoulders, face, and neck. Begin to breathe smoothly, deeply, and rhythmically.

To begin, rest your hands on your thighs with the first finger and thumb lightly pressed together in gyan mudra. You may also practice with the hands in prayer position, anjali mudra, by pressing your palms together at your heart with the thumbs lightly touching just below the sternum. Lightly pull up mula bandha, and keep a gentle lift throughout the entire practice.

Take several slow, deep, and even breaths. Fully exhale all of the breath out.

Inhale through the nose in four equal parts, pausing slightly in between each segment. Keeping a steady beat. Exhale through the nose in four equal parts. Pull your navel into your spine, uddiyana bandha, at each segment.

Start slowly and rhythmically, inhaling in four short segments and exhaling in four short segments, pulling in the navel at each point. Inhale in four parts, exhale in four parts with navel pumps.

As you find a steady rhythm, speed up the pace, building more energy. Keep the breath separated into four distinct parts, briefly pausing in between each segment.

Self

All the love in the infinite universe lies within your heart. Become intimate with the loving rhythms of your heart source. Embrace your love, embrace yourself, and share your love with the world.

Practices and Sequences

Time

Consistency is the most important factor, especially if you want to gain the full benefits of pranayama. Practice every day, without exception.

Practice for several minutes, then pause and rest. Notice how you feel. After a rest, you may resume for two or three more rounds, resting fully in between rounds. When you are ready to complete the practice, lie down and take an extended deep rest. Fully rest for ten minutes or more lying comfortably on your back.

If you are comfortable and would like a faster version of sparkling energy breath, increase the number of segments to seven. Concentrate and make sure you pause completely in between each segment.

Sparkling energy breath is a very energizing and powerful practice, and a little goes a long way. Don't overdo it. Keep your sessions brief and the breathing rhythm steady. Gradually build up the length of your sessions and pace of the breath over time.

Navel Pumping Breath

The abdominal area is home to a confluence of powerful nadis concentrated at your navel center. This area hosts your solar plexus and the third chakra, manipura, linked to the fire element, our sun. A powerful marma point, similar to an acupressure point, called nabhi is located at the navel. It could very well be the most important center in your body for overall health and wellbeing. Before you were born, the navel center provided a portal of nourishment and sustenance while you were inside the womb. It provided your lifeline.

The navel center is responsible for the health of our digestive and nervous systems. An imbalance or blockage in the manipura chakra and surrounding nadis depletes our energy and can cause physical and psychological ailments. If our mind is foggy, or we seem overcome by general feelings of sluggishness, there is often a disturbance in the navel center and weakness in our digestive system.

Pranayamas that utilize uddiyana bandha, navel pumping, stimulate the navel center. This action stokes the digestive fire, and helps us metabolize not only the food we put into our body, but also thoughts, feelings, sensory stimuli, news, internet, environmental events and external circumstances.

This powerful pranayama activates the navel center by strongly pumping the navel multiple times with the breath held out. Make sure to practice on an empty stomach.

Start by coming to a comfortable seated posture with the chest lifted and shoulders and face relaxed. Inhale fully and deeply then exhale completely.

With your breath held out, pump the navel point in and out up to twenty-six times. Keep the chest lifted, shoulders and face relaxed, and spine straight. Each contraction of the navel point also engages the root lock, mula bandha, and each relaxation of the navel point gently releases mula bandha, not fully but just a little bit.

After twenty-six navel pumps, or your capacity, inhale fully and deeply. Exhale completely. Breathe spontaneously for a few breaths, then repeat navel pumping breath for another round. Repeat up to five rounds.

When you are ready to end the practice, lie down and relax deeply for ten minutes. Notice a sense of renewed energy and vigor.

Refine

Slightly widen the nostril tips as you inhale. Develop sensitivity around the inner nostril openings. Subtly entice your gentle breath to waft inward.

Practices and Sequences

Subtle Prana Elevation Breathing

Pull

*Pull up prana
shakti from its
sleepiness in
your root. Pull
it up through all
the vital centers.
Pull it up into
the crown.
Radiate into
infinity.*

This gentle practice works on the subtle layers to softly elevate your prana, your vital life force. The body will remain still while you turn your head slowly from side to side in rhythm with a slow breath and mula bandha. This releases blockages and tension, especially in the upper centers in the chest, neck, face, and skull. Prana rises up into higher energy centers. You can do this practice anywhere, and it is a very effective stress-relieving practice while you are sitting at your office desk or computer.

Sit comfortably in a chair or in a stable posture on the floor. Take several slow, deep, even breaths. Relax your shoulders and face, and make your spine straight and tall. Keep your shoulders wide, try not to round them forward. In this practice, only the head moves. The shoulders, torso, and legs stay still.

To begin, exhale all the breath out of the body. Inhale very slowly as you begin to engage mula bandha and gently turn your head left. Pause slightly and keep mula bandha lifted. Exhale very slowly to the center while relaxing mula bandha just a bit. Pause briefly with the breath held out.

Inhale very, very slowly as you turn your head to the right, pulling up mula bandha. Pause. Exhale very slowly to center, release mula bandha just a little. Pause.

With the head at the center position, inhale very slowly as you gently lift your chin and engage mula bandha. Keep your sternum lifted and chest soft. Shoulders are relaxed. Pause. Release and exhale very slowly to center.

As you breathe in, visualize your vital life force rising up from the base of the body. Your breath and subtle movement is pulling your prana up the spine, removing blockages and stagnation that collects in the lower centers.

Continue this practice for as long as you like. Remember, it is a gentle, but profound practice. Go very, very slowly and breathe softly. You are elevating your prana to nourish the upper centers in your body.

When you are ready to end the practice. Pause, rest and remain quiet and still. Be aware of the light, subtle and pleasant energetic vibrations in your upper centers. Notice that the mind is calm and clear. Enjoy the experience.

Intertwine

Breath and body are interconnected. Breath and mind are interconnected. Breath and emotions are interconnected. Breath and infinity are interconnected.

– Sequences –

When deciding what type of pranayama sequence to practice, it is important to determine your desired intent. Pranayama allows you to control and direct your prana. Do you want an energizing practice? Do you want to neutralize erratic energies and emotions? Or perhaps you are looking to settle and ground. There are infinite combinations of breath techniques, ratios, matras, purakas, rechakas, kumbhakas and bandhas.

You may wish to draw upon the qualities of the three gunas: Rajas, Sattva, Tamas to guide your pranayama practice. Rajasic practices build, expand and amplify pranic energy. Sattvic practices balance, neutralize and soothe. Tamasic practices calm, ground, and slow down the frequency of pranic energy.

Absorb

Allow your mind to become fully consumed with experiencing the movements of consciousness flowing with your breath. Allow your breath to fully absorb you.

Very generally and simply, inhalations energize and exhalations relax. When you want to build energy, lengthen and emphasize inhalations. When you want to calm down and relax, lengthen and emphasize exhalations. The same goes for retentions. Antara kubhaka heightens energy while bahya kubhaka diffuses and suspends pranic energy. Sama pranayamas balance and neutralize energy.

Energizing: Rajasic

Focusing
Natural Breath Awareness 1 minute
Bhastrika (Ego Eradicator) not to exceed 3 minutes
Natural Breath Awareness 1 minute
Repeat above sequence 2 or 3 rounds
Nadi Shodhana 5 minutes

Rejuvenating
Natural Breath Awareness
Ujjayi with Mula Bandha and Uddiyana Bandha on exhale
Bhastrika (Ego Eradicator)
Two Beat Viloma
Natural Breath Awareness

Strengthening, Detoxifying
Natural Breath Awareness
Belly Breathing with Mula Bandha
Slow Bhastrika Right Nostril 1 minute
Slow Bhastrika Left Nostril 1 minute
Slow Bhastrika Both Nostrils 1 minute
Natural Breath Awareness
Repeat 3 rounds

Purifying, Strengthening
Natural Breath Awareness
Kapalbhati
Natural Breath Awareness
Repeat 3 rounds

Uplifting
Natural Breath Awareness
Bhastrika for 20 breaths
Deep three-part breath inhale
Kumbhaka with mula bandha for as long as comfortable
Release bandha and exhale slowly
Repeat 3 times

Balanced Energy
Natural Breath Awareness
Kapalbhati through the right nostril (closing left nostril) 5 breaths
Kapalbhati through the left nostril (closing right nostril) 5 breaths
Deep three-part breath inhale
Kumbhaka
Slowly exhale
Repeat 3 times

Heightened Energy
Keep a steady synchronized rhythm while alternating nostrils after each breath.
Natural Breath Awareness
Full inhale and exhale through the left nostril (closing right)
Full inhale and exhale through the right nostril (closing left)
Full inhale and exhale through the left nostril (closing right)
Full inhale and exhale through the right nostril (closing left)

Proceed

Proceed through life with only the highest most divine pranas in everything you do.

Delicate

Breath is calm when the body is calm. The body is calm when the breath is calm. Be delicate with this. It takes only a flutter of awareness to shift the balance.

Continue for up to three minutes
To end the practice take a full, deep three-part breath inhale
Kumbhaka
Slowly exhale
Repeat 3 times

Balancing and Soothing: Sattvic

Tranquil
Natural Breath Awareness
Belly Breathing
Belly Breathing with Mula Bandha

Calming, Stabilizing
Natural Breath Awareness
Natural Breath Awareness with Arm Movement
3 Part Breath (Yogic Breathing)

Balancing, Focusing
Natural Breath Awareness 3 minutes
Belly Breathing or Ujjayi 3 minutes
Kapalbhati 1 minute
Natural Breath Awareness 2 minutes
Nadi Shodhana 5 minutes

Calming, Focusing, Stabilizing
Natural Breath Awareness
Ujjayi 1:1
Ujjayi 1:2
Ujjayi 1:2:2 with Mula Bandha on retention
Natural Breath Awareness

Calming, Balancing Grounding
Natural Breath Awareness
Nadi Shodhana Left Nostril Only 1:1
Nadi Shodhana Left Nostril Only 1:2
Nadi Shodhana 1:1
Nadi Shodhana 1:2 with Mula Bandha
Natural Breath Awareness

Calming, Soothing
Natural Breath Awareness
Bhramari
Natural Breath Awareness

Tranquil
Natural Breath Awareness
Ujjayi 1:1
Ujjayi 1:2
Ujjayi 1+1:2+2
Natural Breath Awareness

Purifying, Calming, Focusing
Natural Breath Awareness
Bhastrika 1 minute
Inhale through nose count 4
Hold breath in count 7
Exhale through mouth with pursed lips count 8
Repeat 4 cycles
Natural Breath Awareness

Complete
Focusing complete and conscious attention on the flow of inhalation and exhalation, we travel deeper and deeper until we merge with the originating point of all of creation.

Be

*Simply be with
your breath.*

Grounding: Tamasic

Calming, Stabilizing, Grounding
Natural Breath Awareness Lying Down
Natural Breath Awareness in Modified Sphinx
Belly Breathing with Mula Bandha

Balancing and grounding
Begin with 1:1
Then proceed to 1:2:2
Then advance to 1:4:2.
When you have arrived at the ratio 1:4:2, then add external kumbhaka, 1:4:2:2.

Grounding
Natural Breath Awareness
Belly Breathing with Mula Bandha
Ujjayi with Mula Bandha 1:1
Ujjayi with Mula Bandha 1:2
Natural Breath Awareness

Grounding
Natural Breath Awareness
Exhale fully and completely
Bahya Kumbhaka
Inhale fully and completely
Repeat several rounds

Breathing Meditations

*B*reath and the mind are intimately connected. As you breathe slowly, deeply and consciously, meditation will happen all on its own. Pranayama is the bridge between body and mind —it makes meditation accessible. As your mind becomes absorbed in awareness of breath, deep states of meditation can be achieved very gently, easily and naturally.

Expansive Balloon Meditation

This soothing, relaxing meditation is best done lying down in bed, or on the floor. This meditation helps you release emotional and physical density. It can help you expand your perspective, especially during times of stressful challenges in life. It is a nice meditation to do in bed as you drift off to sleep.

Begin by lying down. Make yourself comfortable. If you like, lightly cover yourself with a blanket so you remain warm. Take several slow, deep, and even breaths. Close your eyes and slow down your breath.

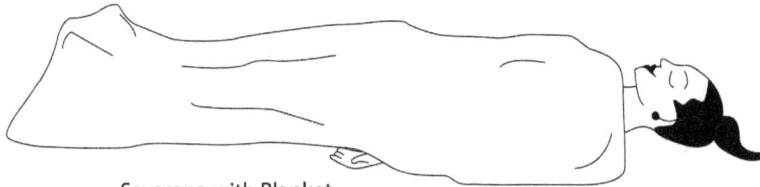

Savasana with Blanket

Become aware of your whole body lying down. Take several breaths simply being aware of your whole body. Observe. Feel. Simply lie still, breathe slowly, and be keenly aware for a few minutes. Feel the weight of your entire body rest on the surface below you. Breathe into the shape of your body. Feel your whole body expand a little as the breath comes in. Feel your whole body deflate just a little as the breath goes out. Stay with this a few moments. Feel your whole body gently expand and yield as the breath flows in. Feel your whole body deflate just a little when the breath leaves.

As breath slowly flows in, imagine your entire body inflating, expanding in all directions, like a balloon in the shape of your body. Begin to lengthen your exhale. As you exhale, keep the feeling of expansion, but allow the body to deflate just a little as the breath flows out. With every inhale, feel the self-balloon grow larger and larger. Keep the sensation of expansion but deflate ever so slightly as you extend the exhalation. Expand and inflate with every inhale. Deflate ever so slightly as you slowly exhale. Continue to inflate yourself to the size of a voluminous balloon. Expand larger than the earth, the sun, our galaxy, the universe. Retain the expansive feelings as you prolong your exhale. Continue to breathe in this way for as long as you like.

Void

Follow your breath to the shunia, to the place where everything dissolves. Float in perfect stillness.

Four-Part Breathing: Empty Bowl Meditation

This pranayama provides an easy, natural introduction to suspending the breath, kumbhaka. This breathing meditation is deeply relaxing, calms the mind, and leads to a quiet, meditative state. Dr. Vasant Lad calls this pranayama, "empty bowl meditation" because, as the breath is suspended in kumbhaka, you become like an empty bowl. Your mind becomes void of thought and you feel a deep sense of tranquility.

Sit comfortably with your palms open and facing up. You may also practice lying down. Close your eyes. If you like, lightly touch the tip of your tongue to the roof of the mouth just behind the front teeth in khechari mudra.

Softly breathe, evenly, and effortlessly. Observe your breath. Simply be aware of the movement of breath. With your eyes closed, direct your attention to the tip of your nose. Be aware of the sensations of air present in the openings of the nostrils. Feel cool air flowing in, and warm air flowing out. Breathe quietly, observing your breath for several minutes.

Next follow the path of your breath. Feel your awareness go with the air into the nose, throat, heart, diaphragm, and deep down into the belly behind the navel, where you will experience a natural pause. Stay in this pause for a brief moment, and then follow the breath as you exhale. Go with your breath as it reverses its path up from the navel behind the diaphragm, heart, throat, through the nostrils, and out of the body, to about nine inches in front of the nose to a second pause.

The first pause is behind the belly button and the second pause is outside the body in space. At these two pauses, breath stops, time stops. Movement of breath is time. In these two pauses, feel that only pure existence is present, divinity is present. Allow yourself to feel suspended in space and time. When the breath stops, you become like an empty bowl. You merge effortlessly and silently into divinity.

Continue slowly. Breathe slowly into your navel and suspend. Breathe out to a point beyond your nostrils and suspend. Release all thoughts.

When you are ready to complete the practice, take a few deep breaths and stretch your arms and legs. Become fully integrated and present in your body, then open your eyes and notice how you feel.

Practice this breathing meditation for ten minutes in the morning and in the evening, and anytime you need a break to calm your mind. Over time, gradually extend the length of your practice. You will find the length of kumbhaka will naturally increase. The feeling of calm and peacefulness will remain with you long after your practice ends.

Chakra Purifying Fountain Breath

This cleansing and energizing meditation is a viloma pranayama with focused awareness at each of the chakra energy centers. You will use a seven-part segmented inhale and a long, flowing exhale.

Surrender

Just as a drop of water merges into oneness with the ocean, surrender the breath from the lungs to become the one cosmic breath that breathes us all.

The chakras are areas of concentrated pranic energy in the body where the nadi channels intersect. Physical, emotional, environmental and spiritual imbalances can lead to congested, weak or blocked flow through the chakras. In chakra purifying breath, we combine focused awareness, conscious breathing and controlled movement of the diaphragm and bandhas to clear blockages and strengthen pranic flow. Chakra purifying breath helps you feel energized, refreshed, clear and aware. You can practice this uplifting breathing meditation as frequently as you like. Purifying and strengthening effects are felt right away for a quick energy surge at the office, home or anytime you feel a bit sluggish or dull.

To begin, find a comfortable seated posture with the spine straight and tall. Close your eyes and rest your hands on your thighs with the thumb and first finger lightly touching in gyan mudra.

As you take several slow, deep breaths visualize and feel into each of the seven chakra centers. Feel into muladhara at the base, swadhisthana just above the pubic bone, manipura at the navel center, anahata at the heart center, vishuddhi at the throat, ajna at the eyebrow center, and sahasrara at the crown. Breathe slowly and deeply for a few moments tuning in to these areas of concentrated energy.

Now lightly engage mula bandha and prepare to start the seven-part inhale. When you are ready, inhale through the nose in seven parts, mindfully pausing at each chakra point then suspending the breath at the crown as you pull up mula bandha. Exhale through the nose and imagine the breath flowing up like a fountain from the crown of the head, then cascading down all around you, enveloping you with vital prana. Pull the breath in from the root and repeat.

Starting from the root, inhale in seven parts, pausing at each chakra center: the perineum, pubic bone, navel, heart, throat pit, eyebrow center, and crown of the head. Retain breath at the crown as mula bandha pulls in a little more. Feel prana rise up from the root to the crown. Then propel the breath up and out of the crown, enveloping yourself with liquid pranic energy as prana cascades all around you and returns back into the base of the body.

Practice this breath meditation for as long as you like. When you are ready to complete the practice, take in a big, deep breath and long hold. Exhale smoothly, then breathe naturally and spontaneously. Pause. Sit or lie down in silence for a while. Be aware of how you feel.

Float

Experience magnificent, transcendent, beauty beyond imagination. Float spontaneously suspended within your blissful breath.

Purifying the Frontal and Spinal Passages Breath

This ancient technique helps you focus your awareness to consciously circulate your prana upward along the front of your body and downward along the back of your body. Along the way, vital prana stimulates and pierces each of your chakra centers in the spine and the corresponding trigger points in the front of the body. The trigger points on the front of the body are called kshetram (SHET-rhum). We can stimulate the chakra centers by focusing conscious awareness into these corresponding trigger points along the front of the body.

Breathing through the frontal and spinal passages is highly soothing, balancing and purifying. This technique has been practiced for thousands of years and forms the basis for many advanced yogic breathing and meditation practices. It helps fos-

Calm

*Breathe in
the essence of
tranquility.*

ter a profound awareness of your subtle pranic energies. It builds concentration, lowers blood pressure, helps eliminate negative or distracting thoughts, and evokes a deep feeling of tranquility and ease.

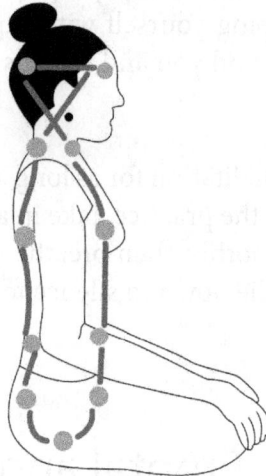

Frontal and Back Passage

To begin, sit up straight and tall. Place your hands gently on your knees. You may lightly touch the first finger and thumb together in gyan mudra if you like. Begin slow, deep and even ujjayi breathing. The tongue may also roll back into khechari mudra.

Slowly feel a stream of prana along the front of your body, like a thin transparent thread, from your navel to the throat pit. This is the frontal passage. Simply breathe using ujjayi and imagine prana being pulled up through a thin tube along the front of the body from the navel center to the throat center as you inhale. Send prana back down from the throat pit to the navel center as you exhale. Continue for several minutes.

Now become aware of a passageway from the eyebrow center, down the back of your spine, and to the root center. Simply breathe using ujjayi, feeling more awareness of prana flowing down from ajna chakra behind the eyebrows, to muladhara chakra in the root. This is the spinal passage. As you inhale, pull prana up from the root through the spine to the eyebrow center. As you exhale, send prana back down from the eyebrow center to the root. Breathe in this way for several minutes.

Now we will begin to circulate our prana up through the frontal passage and down through the spinal passage. We will be aware of the trigger points along the front of the body and chakra centers along the back of the body, but we will keep our breath flowing smoothly. We will not stop and linger at any of the trigger points or chakra centers along the way.

Focus your awareness on muladhara chakra in the base of the body. Slowly inhale and bring your breath up the frontal passage to the throat pit. Be aware of the trigger points at the pubic bone, navel and heart as prana travels up through the frontal passage. Begin to transition to the exhale by bringing awareness from the throat pit to bindu in the back of the skull. Exhale from ajna chakra behind the eyebrows down the spinal passage to vishuddhi chakra in the throat, anahata behind the heart, manipura behind the navel, swadhisthana at the sacrum and back down to muladhara. Slowly inhale up through the frontal passage, and slowly exhale down through the spinal passage.

Allow yourself to feel the invisible, clean and pure stream of pranic energy rise up the front of the body and descend down the back to the root. Be aware that you are sending soothing, purifying prana through each of the trigger points along the frontal passage, and through each of the chakra centers through

Merge

Mind and Prana are intimately connected.

205   *Breathing Meditations*

Transcend

Transcendent Breath: Inhale twenty seconds. Hold twenty seconds. Exhale twenty seconds.

the spinal passage. If you like, you may silently recite a mantra while practicing. Silently repeating "so" on the inhale and "hum" on the exhale is a traditional mantra used in this practice.

Continue for as long as you like. When you are ready to end the practice, begin to breathe spontaneously and naturally. Sit quietly for a good while. Slowly begin to stretch, open your eyes, and be aware of how you feel.

Inner Body Breathing

This breathing meditation allows your awareness to delve deeply into the inner body. It is a gently soothing and profoundly healing practice. As you allow your awareness to flow inside your body, your parasympathetic nervous system becomes more available to help release tension. By increasing conscious awareness of your inner body, you naturally de-stress and soothe your inner systems. Your organs become nourished and supported by your vital life force. Prana can flow smoothly within your inner organs and bodily systems. Breath naturally becomes slow and smooth as your vital organs relax, refresh and restore themselves with healing and vibrant prana. We know that *energy flows where awareness goes*. This meditation trains you to penetrate and bathe specific areas of the body, infusing them with nourishing, healing, positive, life-enhancing prana. Practice inner body breathing for overall well-being, relaxation and health maintenance, or to tune in and send focused healing to weakened or compromised systems and organs.

This meditation best practiced while lying down, but is also effective in any relaxed position. Find a comfortable posture and relax. Breathe slowly, deeply evenly. Extend your exhalations a bit longer than your inhales. Close your eyes and make yourself even more comfortable.

Breathe deeply. Slowly begin to direct your awareness to the softness inside your body. Notice subtle changes in your awareness as you experience the sensations of the outer skin covering your body, and the soft, smooth, moist environment of your inner body. Be with this a while. Breathe and feel into the inner spaces.

Imagine the inner body gently expanding. Feel your organs swell and smoothly begin to move and slide as your breath expands and relaxes your body. Feel your organs softly undulate and glide as gentle waves of breath and fluids move through liquid areas within your body. Feel your navel soften and relax as your belly expands with each incoming breath. Feel waves of breath flow in and around to envelop your organs. Feel steady, rhythmic waves of healing prana flow through your inner body like soft gentle waves washing in with the tide.

Feel your organs gently pulsate, slide and glide and become softer. Allow all of the muscles in your body to soften. Soften the outer surfaces of your organs. Soften the inner tissues. Soften your joints. Soften all of your bones. Soften your outer covering, your skin. Allow softness to permeate your body. Spread this softness out in all directions. Feel all the pores of your skin soften and expand as the entire surface of your skin gently breathes. Breathe deeply. Breathe slowly. Relax.

Feel your body softly rock and sway as the spaces between each organ, tissue, muscle, and joint expand, fully infused with vital pranic energy. Relax. Feel into the areas around your intestines,

Undulate

Experience deep inner pranas undulate peacefully and vibrantly within your body.

bladder, and reproductive organs. Fill them with warm breath, positive fluid energy, and vibrant prana. Linger in this area. Exhale stagnant residues from your body. Feel into your liver, kidneys, pancreas, gallbladder, and adrenals. Fill them with warm liquid breath, positive fluid energy, and vibrancy. Linger here. Exhale stagnant residues from your body. Breathe into your stomach and spleen. Fill them with breath and vitality. Linger here. Exhale stagnant residues from your body. Breathe into and around your lungs. Breathe into the space between the lungs and your ribcage. Fill this entire area with warm breath, positive liquid energy and vibrant prana. Linger. Exhale stagnant residues from your body. Breathe deep into your heart. Feel into your heart and the space around your heart. Fill and embrace this entire area with warm breath, positive fluid energy and vibrant prana. Linger. Exhale stagnant residues from your body. Breathe into your throat and thyroid gland. Soften. Fill this area with warm liquid breath, positive vital energy and vibrant prana. Linger. Exhale stagnant residues from your body. Feel into the areas inside your mouth, inside your face, behind the eyeballs, and deep into the inner ears. Soften. Fill these areas with warm breath, positive fluid energy, and vibrancy. Linger. Exhale stagnant residues from your body. Breathe into and around the brain. Soften. Fill your brain and inner skull with warm vital energy, positive vital energy, and vibrant prana. Linger. Exhale stagnant residues from your body.

Feel and breathe into the entire inner body. Experience the warm, supple inner parts softly pulsate, undulate with each heartbeat and breath. Feel renewed, revitalized, enlivened, and healed. Soften more. Soften your outer covering and feel your skin pulsate with the rhythm of your inner parts. Breathe deeply.

Relax. Rest. Breathe. Observe how you feel.

Breathing into the Five Prana Vayus

These breathing meditations come from Dr. David Frawley, who beautifully describes how to use breath and concentration to develop awareness of the five prana vayus.

Find a comfortable posture for meditation, either seated or reclining. Breathe slowly, deeply and evenly for several moments. Quiet your mind.

Prana Vayu

We will increase awareness of the pranic breath. It is an energizing breath. Take several deep inhalation—imagining drawing prana from the sky and space through the head into the third eye center, ajna chakra. As you exhale, imagine prana emanating from the third eye into all of your senses. Continue for several minutes, bringing prana from sky and space in through the head to the third eye, holding and building prana at the third eye, then exhaling from the eyebrow center, and energizing all of your senses. Bring prana in through the eyes, ears, nostrils, mouth, and mind, purifying the nadis in the head, brain, and sensory organs. As you build energy in the third eye center, feel prana illuminate the inner brain. As you exhale, feel your senses heighten, fully enlivened and purified with prana.

Udana Vayu

We will increase awareness of the uplifting udana breath. Breathe in deeply through the mouth and hold the breath in at the throat chakra, vishuddhi. Loudly project the sound of "om" as you exhale. Breathe in through the mouth into the throat pit, hold and build energy in the throat, then expel the breath with the sound of "om." Imagine sending the vibration of "om" far beyond the horizon and deep into the universe. Continue to practice for as long as you like.

Listen

*Hear the sound
of breath
everywhere.*

Vyana Vayu

We will increase awareness of the expansive, radiant vyana breath. This breathing meditation is best done while standing, but you may practice while seated if you like. Extend your arms wide and bring in a deep, full breath bringing vital energy into your heart and lungs. Keep your arms extended while you retain your breath and imagine sparkling, vital prana radiate from the heart into your blood vessels and spread throughout every cell and atom of your body. Imagine your vital energy radiating out through the hands and feet, traveling far, far away beyond the horizon into deep space. As you exhale, close your arms and bring your hands together at the heart center in anjali mudra, prayer hands. Imagine that your heart is the center of all energy, of all creation. Continue for as long as you like.

Samana Vayu

We will increase awareness of the centering, balancing samana breath. Take a few silent moments to imagine the entire cosmos. Imagine feeling energy from all the galaxies, stars, and planets. Draw energy from the entire cosmos deep into your body. Deeply inhale this universal energy into your navel center, fueling the digestive fire. Hold your breath and send energy into the navel, feeling the digestive fire heat up and burn brightly. As you exhale, send this bright energy swirling outward through all of the muscles, tissues, and organs, nourishing every cell and atom of your body. Continue for as long as you like.

Apana Vayu

We will increase awareness of the grounding, stabilizing apana breath. This practice is best done while seated with your feet firmly placed on the ground. Draw in a slow, deep breath, bringing pranic energy down into the base of your spine. Imagine your body is a giant, heavy stone mountain. Hold your breath at the base of the spine, feeling stable and secure like a mountain. Exhale and send your energy downward through your legs and feet, releasing all physical and mental toxins and residues deep down into the earth. Continue for as long as you like.

All Five Pranas
Practice the vayu meditations in sequence, ten breaths each, beginning with prana, udana, vyana, samana, and apana. Continue for ten breaths each in reverse order, with apana, samana, vyana, udana then prana.

So Hum Breath Meditation

"When sound, breath, and awareness come together, it becomes light... So Hum meditation properly practiced leads to the union of the individual with the universal Cosmic Consciousness. You will go beyond thought, beyond time and space, beyond cause and effect. Limitations will vanish."– Dr. Vasant Lad

So Hum is a breathing meditation using a mantra that has been used since ancient times. So Hum is a profound, yet simple practice. It is soothing, relaxing and balancing, and it improves concentration. It works deeply on the subtle prana layers, and brings about a sense of unity, love, and grace. It is very easy to practice and is often recommended for people just beginning to learn to meditate.

So Hum is said to be the sound of life, the sound of nature, the sound of prana – the sound of breath. All living things breathe, and the sound of So Hum exists inside the breath of all living things. *So* is the sound of the inhale and *Hum* is the sound of the exhale. When we practice the So Hum breath meditation, we are

Mind

Pranayama is only possible with focused concentration and alert engagement of your mind.

feeling our divine connection to all of life. So Hum is translated as *"I am That."* As we practice so hum breathing meditation, we allow ourselves to merge with the flow of the universal cosmos.

To practice So Hum meditation, silently say "Soooooooooooo" as the breath comes in and "Hummmmmmmmm" as the breath flows out. So Hum can be practiced in any posture.

To begin, make yourself comfortable and begin slow, deep, steady breathing. You may wish to use a very gentle ujjayi breath. Close your eyes and increase your awareness of breath flowing in from your nostrils, through your throat down to your navel. Be aware of your breath flowing back out from your navel up through your throat and out through your nostrils. Breath is conscious, deep and slow. Try to breathe in such a way that there is no disturbance in the nasal membranes and throat passage. Imagine the breath flowing gently through the center of your airways with no friction along the sides.

Now begin to introduce the mantra, synchronizing the So Hum mantra with the breath. Silently say "Soooooooooooo" the full length of your inhale, and "Hummmmmmmmm" the full length of your exhale. Make your breath smooth. Breathe in So and breathe out Hum. Remain continuously aware of the mantra So Hum as the breath flows in and out. Feel increasingly aware of very subtle vibrations as the internal sounds so and hum are heard within.

Continue the So Hum breath meditation for as long as you like. When you feel complete and are ready to end the practice, become aware and fully present in your body. Breathe spontaneously and naturally. Become fully aware of your surroundings. Take time to pause for a little while and rest. Notice how you feel.

Pranic Regeneration

We lose prana through daily activities and stress. Vital health is dependent upon a sufficient quantum of prana and pranic reserves. We don't want to deplete our prana because that is when we weaken, become fatigued, run down, and lose our vigor. It is important to recharge our pranic energies, build more prana, and create a pranic reserve.

In this meditation, we learn to pull in more prana, build pranic energy, then consciously distribute prana, directing pranic energy into specific areas of the body. We begin to develop prana vidya, a deeper knowledge of prana and ability to manipulate the flow of pranic energy.

This meditation can be practiced either sitting or lying down, just make sure the spine is very straight. Close your eyes, or keep them very slightly open and gaze at the tip of the nose in nasik-agra drishti. Begin slow, steady, deep breathing.

Begin to focus your concentration on the nostrils. As you inhale, feel that you are building prana inside the nasal passages. Begin to feel prana penetrate into the nostrils. Feel more energy in the nostrils and begin to feel the nostrils absorb pure pranic energy. Stay with this awhile. Absorb more pranic energy through the nostrils. Keep your breath steady and slow. Concentrate your awareness on building prana inside the nostrils. Feel the nostril linings absorb more pranic energy. You are bringing more prana into the body. You are increasing the quantum of prana in your body. If you like, visualize the pranic energy as pure light penetrating into the linings of the nostrils. You may also silently say a mantra. "Om," "So Hum," or "Sat Nam" are mantras you may want to incorporate here.

Shakti

Energize every atom in your body with vital pranic energy.

Now take a slow, deep breath, accumulating more prana in your nostrils. Close your eyes, and retain the breath. Apply mula bandha and jalandhara bandha. Concentrate your awareness in the navel region. Send pranic energy to the area of the navel. Begin to increase the pranic energy you feel inside the abdomen around your navel area. Build it up, charge it up. You may visualize the prana as bright light getting more intense. Hold your breath in for as long as comfortable, but don't overdo it. You will need to exhale for a long period of time, so make sure you don't retain your breath for too long.

You will now very, very slowly exhale and distribute your prana. You may choose to focus your prana on a particular area of the body that needs more energy or healing, or allow your prana to diffuse throughout your entire body. Really concentrate. Visualize prana as warm, liquid light if you like.

Repeat several times. Build prana in the nostril linings. Inhale it deeply inside the body to the navel. Retain your breath as prana builds and charges up. Concentrate and slowly, slowly exhale as you distribute concentrated prana throughout the body or to a specific part.

When you are ready to end the practice, relax and breathe slowly and naturally. Rest and absorb the benefits of your meditation.

Marma Breathing Meditation

"One should practice concentration by drawing one's Prana by the power of attention from each of these marma regions." Vasishta Samhita, ancient yogic Veda

This guided meditation is designed to help you consciously focus awareness, breath, and vibrant prana into specific points on your body to bring about healing, greater clarity, vitality, purification, and radiant beauty. The Vedic term for this process is prana chikitsa, or pranic healing. The yogis identified important, sensitive pressure points on the body, much like acupressure or acupuncture points. These points on the surface of the body connect to the nadi channels and chakra centers and may be manipulated by touch, mantra, light, and even gemstones to send concentrated prana to specific areas of the body for profound healing. In this meditation, we use our concentration and breathing to build up a charge of concentrated prana at specific marma points, bathing the nearby area with vital prana.

Dr. David Frawley explains there are eighteen marma points on the body classically used to draw energized prana inward into the body for healing and purification. In this practice you will concentrate your awareness and prana in each of these specific points starting with the feet. You will focus your attention and breathing on one region then on to another, ascending from the bottom of the body to the top. Finally, you will hold your awareness, and breath, at the top of the head. As you become familiar with the marma point breathing, you can use this process to direct your breath and attention to any area of your body to heal, renew, and purify.

Begin the practice by coming into a comfortable position, either lying down or sitting. Keep your spine straight and situate yourself so that you will be comfortable and still. Close your eyes and begin to direct your attention to the flow of your breath. Breathe slowly, smoothly and evenly with a soft ujjayi breath. Relax as you hear the soft, gentle sound of your breath coming in and out of your body. Feel your breath flow smoothly.

Positive

Breathe in and out through every Pore of your skin.

215 *Breathing Meditations*

Stimulate

Vibrate vital prana into bright points of light throughout your body.

Begin to focus on the path of your breath as it flows in through the nostrils and travels deep into the belly. Observe your breath flow up through your nostrils and out of your body. Observe your breath flow in, deep into the body then out again for a few moments.

Keep a long, smooth, slow and steady rhythm to your breath and begin to develop greater awareness of your body. Feel your whole body from the soles of your feet to the top of your head. Begin to feel your whole body expand as you inhale. Feel the whole body relax and slightly deflate as you exhale. Breathe in and feel your body expand. Breathe out and feel your body deflate. Feel a sense of stillness and calm, and begin to become aware of your entire body settling into stillness. Be aware of your body and be aware of complete stillness within your body.

Send awareness to your toes. On inhalation, gather concentrated energy into your toes. As you exhale, release the energy. Feel vibrancy in your toes. Feel your toes energized, relaxed and rejuvenated.

Draw focused attention up to your ankles. On inhalation, gather concentrated energy in your ankles. On exhalation, release it. Feel vibrancy in your ankles. Feel your ankles energized, relaxed and rejuvenated.

Draw focused attention up to the middle of your calves. On inhalation, gather concentrated energy there. On exhalation, release it. Feel vibrancy in the middle of your calves. Feel your calves energized, relaxed and rejuvenated.

Draw focused attention up to the base of your knees. On inhalation, gather concentrated energy in the base of your knees. On exhalation, release it. Feel vibrancy in the base of your knees. Feel this area energized, relaxed and rejuvenated.

Bring awareness up to the middle of your knees. On inhalation, gather concentrated energy in the middle of your knees. On exhalation, release it. Feel vibrancy in the middle of your knees. Feel this area energized, relaxed and rejuvenated.

Move your energy up to the middle of your thighs. On inhalation, gather concentrated energy in the middle of your thighs. On exhalation, release it. Feel vibrancy in the middle of your thighs. Feel this area energized, relaxed and rejuvenated.

Send your energy up to the root of the anus. On inhalation, gather concentrated energy at your anus. On exhalation, release it. Feel vibrancy here. Feel this area energized, relaxed and rejuvenated.

Bring awareness up to the middle of your hips. On inhalation, gather concentrated energy in the middle of your hips. On exhalation, release it. Feel vibrancy in your hips. Feel this area energized, relaxed and rejuvenated.

Bring awareness up to the root of your urethra. On inhalation, gather concentrated energy in the root of your urethra. On exhalation, release it. Feel vibrancy here. Feel this area energized, relaxed and rejuvenated.

Move your energy to your navel. On inhalation, gather concentrated energy in the navel. On exhalation, release it. Feel vibrancy in the navel. Feel this area energized, relaxed and rejuvenated.

Infuse

Permeate your body, mind and soul with vibrant prana.

Breathing Meditations

Evolve

Ascend into vibrant, radiant life force energy.

Send your energy up to your heart. On inhalation, gather concentrated energy in your heart. On exhalation, release it. Feel vibrancy here. Feel your heart area energized, relaxed and rejuvenated.

Send energy up to the base of your throat. On inhalation, gather concentrated energy in the base of your throat. On exhalation, release it. Feel vibrancy here. Feel this area energized, relaxed and rejuvenated.

Bring awareness up to the root of your tongue. On inhalation, gather concentrated energy in the root of your tongue. On exhalation, release it. Feel vibrancy here. Feel the root of your tongue energized, relaxed and rejuvenated.

Bring awareness up to the root of your nose. On inhalation, gather concentrated energy in the root of your nose. On exhalation, release it. Feel vibrancy here. Feel the root of your nose energized, relaxed and rejuvenated.

Move your energy up to your eyes. On inhalation, gather concentrated energy in your eyes. On exhalation, release it. Feel vibrancy here. Feel your eyes energized, relaxed and rejuvenated.

Move your energy up to the point between your eyebrows. On inhalation, gather concentrated energy there. On exhalation, release it. Feel vibrancy between your eyebrows. Feel this area of your body energized, relaxed and rejuvenated.

Bring your energy up to the middle of the forehead. On inhalation, gather concentrated energy in the middle of your forehead. On exhalation, release it. Feel vibrancy here. Feel the center of your forehead energized, relaxed and rejuvenated.

Send concentrated energy up to the crown of your head. On inhalation, gather concentrated energy at the top of your head. On exhalation, release it. Feel vibrancy here. Feel the top of your head energized, relaxed and rejuvenated.

Take a big, deep breath from your toes all the way up to the top of your head. Focus your energy and concentration at the crown of your head while you hold the breath in. Feel your pranic energy expand throughout your body as you retain your breath at the crown. Slowly exhale all of your breath out. Lie still and rest for as long as you like.

When you are ready to end the practice, keep your eyes closed and begin to breathe naturally and spontaneously. Begin to hear the sounds in the room around you, and become more aware of your whole body. Feel energy in your hands, your feet, your arms, your legs, your hips, your torso, your shoulders, your neck, and your head. Feel your whole body. Be fully aware of all of the sensations in your body and be fully aware of your physical surroundings.

When you feel you are ready, very slowly begin to bring gentle movement into the body. Wiggle your fingers, wiggle your toes, stretch your arms up over your head, and stretch your legs. Slowly open your eyes and end the practice.

Radiant Heart Breathing

This beautiful breathing meditation helps you deeply relax and gently purify and cleanse the energetic pathways associated with your heart center. The heart center, anahata chakra is linked to

Treasure

Place hands in open bowl mudra... palms open, lightly cupped, pinky fingers and outer edges of hands together, elbows resting alongside ribs. Breathe deeply into the golden treasure of your heart.

Breathing Meditations

Heal

Feel your prana radiate with every vibrant, healing pulsation of your heartbeat.

our feelings, emotions, and deep experiences of pure and unconditional love, beauty, compassion, acceptance, and understanding.

Sit or lie down quietly in any comfortable position with your eyes closed. If you are lying down, cover yourself with a blanket so you remain warm during the practice. Become still and comfortable, yet awake and alert. If you are sitting in a chair, keep your feet securely on the floor and feel your buttocks balanced evenly. Establish a feeling of stability and become aware of your entire body. Feel secure and grounded. Sense a slight heaviness in your tail bone and at the same time become aware of a sensation of lightness at the crown of your head. Breathe comfortably and naturally.

Relax your arms and hands. Situate your palms so that they are facing up. Be comfortable. If you like, you may wish to place your hands in a mudra called hridaya mudra while doing this heart-opening practice. This mudra facilitates channeling prana into the heart.

For hridaya mudra, place the tips of the index fingers at the root of the thumbs. Then very gently press the tips of the thumbs into the tips of the middle and ring fingers. The pinkie finger stays straight and the palms face upward. Close your eyes, be still, and breathe comfortably and naturally.

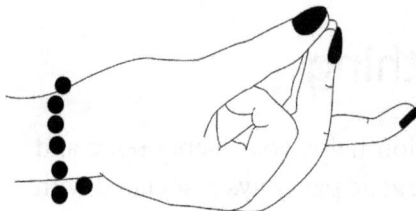

Hridya Mudra

Now direct your attention to the area of your heart. Breathe slowly, deeply, evenly. Imagine that center of your heart is the source point for all of the love in the universe. You may want to imagine a soothing color or peaceful image here.

*Breathe into the
infinite wisdom
of your heart.*

As you inhale slowly, imagine your breath coming in from all directions into your heart. Visualize your breath flowing in through every pore on the surface of your skin, deeply into the very core of your heart. Feel your heart center become warm and glowing. As you exhale slowly, send your breath out through the pores of your skin, out in all directions from the center point of your heart.

Continue imagining and feeling your breath flow in from all directions through the pores of your skin deep into your heart center, then radiate out in every direction. Slowly inhale and draw the breath in through your skin deeper and deeper into a brilliant, radiant point at center of your heart. Gently, slowly exhale, and feel your glowing breath radiate out in all directions far away into the distance.

With each inhale and exhale, you will feel more spacious and relaxed. Feel unconditional love penetrate every cell of your body. Continue for a while longer. As you become more relaxed and comfortable, feel the brilliant warm glow of the light deep within your heart space. Linger here.
Smoothly exhale, imagine this warm glowing light traveling outward in every direction, carried by your breath. Send it as far away as it can travel. Pause.

Breathe into the brilliant point of light deep within your heart. Pause. Gently and smoothly release your breath out as far away as you can imagine, out beyond the stars into the farthest reaches of the cosmos. Pause.

Gather your breath back in, and feel it flow deep into the center of your heart. Pause.

Wonder

Breath provides a divine environment for infinite manifestation.

Continue to softly breathe deeply into a very brilliant fine point within your heart, then softly radiate, exhaling into the vast distance.

Imagine your breath drawing deeper and deeper into the core of your heart as you inhale and pause, and imagine sending your breath farther and farther away into the distance as you exhale and pause.

As your meditation feels complete, begin to breathe normally and naturally. Become fully aware of your physical body and notice any changes in awareness or sensations. Continue to lie still and begin to feel a sense of warmth and vibrancy in the palms of your hands and the soles of your feet. Then allow this sense of warmth and vibrancy begin to spread into the legs and arms, into the torso, neck and head.

Very slowly and softly, begin to bring gentle movement into your toes and fingers. Begin to breathe more actively, stretch your arms up over your head, and stretch your toes away from your fingertips.

When you feel fully present and grounded, very slowly begin to open your eyes. Sit up quietly, straight and tall, as you become fully aware of your body and your physical surroundings. Notice any changes or sensations that you may be feeling. Stretch and move your body, complete the practice, and smile.

Glossary

Agni (AHG-nee) Fire element

Ajna Chakra (AHGN-yah) Pranic energy center associated with the pineal gland and located at the third eye, in the brain at the eyebrow center

Akasha (ah-KAH-shah) Ether or space element

Amrit (UM-rit) Divine nectar

Anahata Chakra (ah-NAH-hah-tuh) Pranic energy center associated with the heart, located in the chest

Anandamaya Kosha (AH-nun-duh-my-uh) (KOH-shuh) Energetic sheath of bliss, infinite heart

Annamaya Kosha (AH-nah-my-uh) (KOH-shuh) Energetic sheath of the physical body, food body

Antara Kumbhaka (AN-ta-ruh) (KOOM-bha-kuh) Holding the breath in; internal breath retention

Anuloma Viloma (ah-noo-LOHM-uh) (vee-LOHM-uh). Anuloma means in the right direction, and viloma means in the opposite direction. Alternate nostril breathing technique also called nadi shodhana.

Apana Vayu (u-PAH-nuh) (VAH-EE-oo) Downward moving energy; sub-prana moving downward from the navel to perineum responsible for elimination and reproduction

Apas (AH-pas) Water element

Asana (AH-sah-nuh) Yoga pose; steady and comfortable meditative posture

Bandha (BUN-duh) Yogic energy lock or hold

Bhairava Mudra (by-RHAH-vuh) (MOO-dhruh) Left hand is placed in the right with both palms facing up and both hands resting in the lap. Mudra representing ida and pingala nadis used in pranayama and meditation.

Bhastrika (bah-STREE-kah) Bellows breath or breath of fire; a rapid vigorous pranayama

Bhaya Kumbhaka (BHY-uh) (KOOM-bha-kuh) Holding the breath out; external breath retention

Bhramari (BHRAH-mah-ree) Bee; humming bee pranayama

Bindu (BIN-doo) Dot or point of concentrated energy. Sacred symbol of the center of creation, and entire cosmos in the unmanifest state. Important energetic point at the upper back of skull similar to a chakra.

Chakra (CHAH-krah) Wheel, circle or vortex of concentrated pranic energy in the subtle body; conglomeration point of nadi channels

Chandra (CHAHN-druh) Moon

Chandra Bhedana (CHAHN-druh) (BHEH-duh-nuh) Left nostril breathing; from chandra, moon and bhedana, pass through. Activates ida nadi

Chitta (CHI-tuh) Individual mind including consciousness, subconscious and unconscious aspects of mind

Gunas (GOO-nus) Three qualities of nature; rajas, tamas, sattwa

Ida (EE-duh) Left nostril or lunar nadi, associated with internal awareness

Jalandhara Bandha (JAH-lan-dhah-ruh) (BUN-duh) Throat or chin lock

Kapalbhati (KAH-p-hal-bhah-tee) Shining skull breath; energizing pranayama; one of the six traditional shatkarmas or yogic cleansing practices

Kevala Kumbaka (KHE-vuh-luh) KOOM-bha-kuh) Naturally arising, spontaneous breath retention resulting from deep bliss, samadhi

Khechari Mudra (KEH-cha-ree) (MOO-dhruh) Tongue mudra performed by rolling tip of tongue back to touch the upper palate

Kshetram (SHET-rhum) Trigger points along the front of the body to activate individual chakras

Kosha (KOH-shuh) Energetic sheath of the subtle energy body

Kumbhaka (KOOM-bha-kuh) Breath retention

Kundalini Shakti (koon-duh-LEE-nee) (SHAHK-tee) Potential vital life force energy dormant in the base of the spine

Manipura Chakra (mah-nee-POOR-ruh) (CHAH-krah) Pranic energy center associated with the navel center, solar plexus, located behind the navel

Manomaya Kosha (mah-NOH-my-uh) (KOH-shuh) Energetic sheath of the mental body

Marma (MAR-muh) Energetically sensitive points on the body

Matra (MAH-truh) Unit of time, beat or rhythm; syllable of mantra

Mantra (MAHN-truh) Sound vibration used to activate energy

Mula Bandha (MOO-luh) (BUN-duh) Root lock

Muladhara Chakra (MOO-lah-dhah-ruh) (CHAH-krah) Pranic energy center in the base of the body, located in the perineum

Nabhi (NAH-bhee) Powerful marma point at the navel

Nadi (NAH-dee) Flow, channels of pranic energy in the subtle body

Nadi Shodhana (NAH-dee) (SHO-dha-nuh) Alternate nostril breathing; cleansing and balancing nadi channels

Pancha Vayu (PAHN-chah) (VAH-EE-oo) Five vital airs, directional movements of pranic energy felt and located in the physical body; the human experience of pranic sensation in the body

Pingala (PEEN-gah-luh) Right nostril or solar nadi, associated with external awareness

Prana (PRAH-nah) Vital life energy permeating entire cosmos

Prana Shakti (PRAH-nah) (SHAHK-tee) Powerful force of vital energy, solar life-supporting energy

Prana Vayu (PRAH-nah) (VAH-EE-oo) Sub-prana moving upwards in the chest region; controls lungs and heart

Prana (PRAH-nah) (VID-yuh) Knowledge of prana, and resulting ability to consciously manipulate prana

Pranamaya Kosha (PRA-nah-my-uh) (KOH-shuh) Energetic sheath of prana or vital energy body

Pranayama (prah-nah-YAH-muh) Expansion of the dimensions of prana, vital life force, through series of techniques

Puraka (POO-ra-kuh) Inhalation

Rajas (RAH-jahs) One of the three gunas; quality in nature of activity, passion, agitation

Rechaka (REH-chuh-kuh) Exhalation

Sahasrara Chakra (sah-hah-SRAH-ruh) (CHAH-krah) Pranic energy center at the crown of the head, associated with the pituitary gland, seat of high consciousness

Samadhi (sa-MAH-dhee) Blissful state of self-realization

Sama Vritti (SAH-mah) (VRIT-hee) Same breath, inhalation and exhalation are equal duration. Sama is same and vritti is movement or fluctuation

Samana Vayu (suh-MAH-nuh) (VAH-EE-oo) Balancing sub-prana moving sideways and inward in the abdominal region; controls digestion and assimilation

Samskara (sam-SKAH-ruh) Deep-seated motivation; habit

Sattwa (SAHT-wuh) One of the three gunas; quality in nature of balance, harmony, purity

Shambhavi Mudra (sham-BHAH-vhee) (MOO-dhruh) Eyebrow centering gazing; mudra that awakens pineal gland and ajna chakra.

Simhasana (sim-HA-sah-nuh) Lion pose; energizing cleansing pranayama technique

Sitali (SEE-tah-lee) Cooling breath; pranayama using curled tongue to cool breath

Sitkari (SEET-kah-ree) Hissing breath; pranayama using rush of air around teeth to cool breath

Surya (SOOR-yuh) Sun

Surya Bhedana (SOOR-yuh) (BHEH-duh-nuh) Right nostril breathing; from surya, sun and bhedana, pass through. Activates pingala nadi

Sushumna (soo-SHOOM-nuh) Main, central nadi in the center of the spinal cord

Shunia (SHOON-yuh) Void

So Hum (SOH) (HUM) Cosmic, universal sound current in breath; mantra for breath; 'I am That'

Swadhisthana Chakra (swah-dhi-STAH-nuh) (CHAH-krah) Pranic energy center at the sacrum, associated with the sacral plexus

Tamas (TAH-mas) One of the three gunas; quality in nature of inertia, dullness, sluggishness

Udana Vayu (oo-DAH-nuh) (VAH-EE-oo) Upwards moving energy; sub-prana moving upwards in the head, arms and legs

Uddiyana Bandha (OO-dee-ah-nah) (BUN-duh) Abdominal lock; 'flying up'

Ujjayi (OO-jay) Victorious Breath; throat breath; soothing, energizing pranayama

Vijnanamaya Kosha (vig-NAH-nuh-my-uh) (KOH-shuh) Energetic sheath of knowledge, intuition, wisdom energy body

Glossary

Viloma (vee-LOH-muh) Against the grain; against the hair; interrupted flow pranayama

Vishuddhi Chakra (vih-SHOO-dhuh) (CHAH-krah) Pranic energy center at the throat pit, associated with the thyroid gland and cervical plexus

Vyana Vayu (vee-YAH-nuh) (VAH-EE-oo) Expansive vital force; sub-prana pervading the entire body

Bibliography

Anderson, Sandra; Solvik, Rolf. *Yoga Mastering the Basics*. Honesdale, PA: The Himalayan Institute Press, 2000.

Bachman, Nicolai. *The Language of Ayurveda*. Victoria, BC, Canada: Trafford Publishing, 2006.

Beauchaine, Theodore. "Vagal Tone, Development and Gray's Motivational Theory: Toward an Integrated Model of Autonomic Nervous System Functioning in Psychopathology." *Development and Psychopathology*, vol. 13, no. 2, pp. 183-214, 2001.

Bhajan, Yogi. *The Aquarian Teacher: KRI International Teacher Training in Kundalini Yoga as taught by Yogi Bhajan Level 1 Instructor Textbook*. Espanola, New Mexico: Kundalini Research Institute, 2007.

Bhajan, Yogi. *The Aquarian Teacher: KRI International Teacher Training in Kundalini Yoga as taught by Yogi Bhajan Level 1 Instructor Manual*. Espanola, New Mexico: Kundalini Research Institute, 2010.

Buddhananda, Swami. *Moola Bandha The Master Key*. Munger, Bihar, India: Yoga Publications Trust, Bihar School of Yoga, 1978.

Calais-Germain, Blandine. *Anatomy of Breathing*. Seattle, WA: Eastland Press, 2006.

Desikachar, T.K.V. *The Heart of Yoga: Developing a Personal Practice*. Rochester, Vermont: Inner Traditions International, 1995.

Dhruva A, et al. "Yoga Breathing for Cancer Chemotherapy-Associated Symptoms and Quality of Life: Results of a Pilot Randomized Controlled Trial." *Journal of Alternative and Complementary Medicine.*18 (5):473-9, May 2012.

Farhi, Donna. *The Breathing Book: Good Health and Vitality through Essential Breath Work*. New York: St. Martins Press, 1996.

Farhi, Donna. *Yoga Mind, Body and Spirit: A Return to Wholeness.* New York: Holt, 2000.

Frawley, David. *Ayurveda and the Mind.* Twin Lakes, WI: Lotus Press, 1996.

Frawley, David. *Mantra Yoga and Primal Sound: Secret of Seed (Bija) Mantras.* Twin Lakes, WI: Lotus Press, 2010.

Frawley, David. *Yoga & Ayurveda: Self-Healing and Self-Realization.* Twin Lakes, WI: Lotus Press, 1999.

Frawley, David; Ranade, Subhash; Lele, Avinash. *Ayurveda and Marma Therapy: Energy Points in Yogic Healing.* Twin Lakes, WI: Lotus Press, 2003.

Hanh, Thich Nhat. *Breathe, You Are Alive: Sutra on the Full Awareness of Breathing.* Berkeley, CA: Parallax Press, 2008.

Hayama Yuka, Inoue Tomoko. "The Effects of Deep Breathing on 'Tension–Anxiety' and Fatigue in Cancer Patients Undergoing Adjuvant Chemotherapy." *Complementary Therapies in Clinical Practice,* Vol. 18, Issue 2, p94–98. Published online: November 11, 2011.

Hendricks, Gay. *Conscious Breathing: Breathwork for Health, Stress Release and Personal Mastery.* Bantam Books, 1995.

Hewitt, James. *Complete Yoga Book, The Yoga of Breathing, the Yoga of Posture, and the Yoga of Meditation.* New York: Shocken Books, 1977.

Iyengar, B.K.S. *Light on Life: The Yoga Journey to Wholeness, Inner Peace and Ultimate Freedom.* Rodale Books, 2005.

Iyengar, B.K.S. *Light on Pranayama: The Yogic Art of Breathing.* New York: Crossroad Publishing, 1999.

Khalsa, Harijot Kaur. *Praana, Praanee, Praanayam, Exploring the Breath Technology of Kundalini Yoga as Taught by Yogi Bhajan.* Espanola, New Mexico: Kundalini Research Institute, 2006.

Khalsa, Shakti Parwha Kaur. *Kundalini Yoga: The Flow of Eternal Power. A Simple Guide to the Yoga of Awareness. New York: Perigee Books, 1996.*

Kilham, Christopher. *The Five Tibetans.* Rochester, VT: Healing Arts Press, 1994.

Lad, Dr. Vasant. *Ayurveda the Science of Self-Healing.* Twin Lakes WI: Lotus Press, 1985.

Lad, Dr. Vasant. *The Complete Book of Ayurvedic Home Remedies.* New York: Three Rivers Press, 1998.

Lad, Dr. Vasant; Durve, Anisha. *Marma Points of Ayurveda: the Energy Pathways for Healing Body, Mind and Consciousness with a Comparison to Traditional Chinese Medicine.* Twin Lakes WI: Lotus Press, 1985.

Lewis, Dennis. *Free Your Breath, Free Your Life: How Conscious Breathing Can Relieve Stress, Increase Vitality, and Help You Live More Fully.* Boston: Shambhala Press, 2004.

Muktibodhananda, Swami. *Hatha Yoga Pradipika.* Bihar School of Yoga. Munger, Bihar, India: Yoga Publications Trust, Bihar School of Yoga, 1998.

Niranjananda Saraswati, Swami. *Prana Pranayama Prana Vidya.* Munger, Bihar, India: Bihar School of Yoga, Swami Satyasangananda Saraswati, 1994.

Rama, Swami; Ballentine, Rudolph; Hymes, Alan. *Science of Breath A Practical Guide.* Honesdale, PA: Himalayan Institute, 1979.

Rosen, Richard. *Pranayama beyond the Fundamentals: An Indepth Guide to Yogic Breathing.* Boston: Shambhala, 2006.

Rosen, Richard. *The Yoga of Breath: A Step-by-Step Guide to Pranayama.* Boston: Shambhala, 2002.

Satyasangananda, Swami. *Tattwa Shuddhi: The Tantric Practice of Inner Purification.* Munger, Bihar, India: Yoga Publications Trust, Bihar School of Yoga, 1984.

Satyananda Saraswati, Swami. *Asana Pranayama Mudra Bandha.* Munger, Bihar, India: Yoga Publications Trust, Bihar School of Yoga, 1969.

Satyananda Saraswati, Swami. *Kundalini Tantra.* Munger, Bihar, India: Yoga Publications Trust, Bihar School of Yoga, 1984.

Satyananda Saraswati, Swami. *Four Chapters on Freedom: Commentary on Yoga Sutras of Patanjali.* Munger, Bihar, India: Yoga Publications Trust, Bihar School of Yoga, 1976.

Satyananda Saraswati, Swami. *A Systematic Course in the Ancient Tantric Techniques of Yoga and Kriya.* Munger, Bihar, India: Yoga Publications Trust, Bihar School of Yoga, 1981.

Scaravelli, Vanda. *Awakening the Spine.* Switzerland: Labyrinth Publishing S.A., 1991.

Schiffmann, Erich, *Yoga the Spirit and Practice of Moving Into Stillness.* New York: First Pocket Books, 1996.

Sharma, Sachin; Telles, Shirley; Balkrishna, Acharya. "Effect of Alternate Nostril Yoga Breathing on Autonomic and Respiratory Variables." *Indian Journal of Physiology and Pharmacology*, vol. 55, No. 5.

Sivananda, Swami. *Kundalini Yoga*. Tehri-Garhwal, Uttarakhand, India: The Divine Life Society, 1935.

Telles, Shirley; Desiraju, T. "Heart Rate Alterations in Different Types of Pranayamas." *Indian Journal of Physiology and Pharmacology, 36 (4): 287-288, 1992.*

Telles, Shirley, Nagarathna, R; Nagendra, H.R. "Breathing through a Particular Nostril can Alter Metabolism and Autonomic Activities." *Indian Journal of Physiology and Pharmacology,* 38(2): 133-137, 1994.

Upadhyay, Dhungel; Malhotra, V; Sarkar, D; Prajapati, R. "Effect of Alternate Nostril Breathing Exercise on Cardiorespiratory Functions." *Nepal Med Coll Journal,* 10:25–27, 2008.

Weil, Andrew. *Breathing: the Master Key to Self-Healing.* Sounds True. 1999.

Van Lysebeth, Andre. *Pranayama: The Yoga of Breathing. United Kingdom: Harmony Publishing, 1983.*

Vernon, Rama Jyoti. *Yoga: The Practice and Myth of Sacred Geometry.* Twin Lakes, WI: Lotus Press, 2014.

Resources

Resources

www.ayurveda.com
Dr. Vasant Lad

www.bigshakti.com
Dr. Swami Shankardev Saraswati and Jayne Stevenson

www.biharyoga.net
Home Page for Satyananda yoga and Bihar yoga

www.drsvoboda.com
Dr. Robert Svoboda

www.pranavinyasaflow.com
Shiva Rea

www.vedanet.com
Dr. David Frawley (Vamadeva)

www.3ho.org
Yogi Bhajan

About the Author

Deborah Garland, MA, CAS, PKT, E-RYT 500, is a clinical Ayurveda practitioner, Panchakarma Specialist, yoga instructor, author and herbalist in Paradise Valley, AZ where she has taught pranayama and yoga for over 25 years. Deborah is the author of 365 Ways To Breathe, and Ayurveda: How to Live a Vibrantly Radiant Life. She is the creator and formulator of Eternal Radiance Ayurveda Organic Ayurveda products. She works with individual clients, teaches classes and workshops and hosts retreats. Her specialty is helping people make small, easy to manage adjustments in lifestyle to make positive shifts in physical, emotional and spiritual wellness through Ayurveda, Yoga and Vedic Counseling. Everyone she works with learns Self-Healing techniques from Ayurveda, pranayama, yoga and universal wellness principles. Whether teaching a yoga class, working with someone affected by dis-ease, leading a seminar or retreat, or facilitating pranayama and meditation, her focus is the same: helping people feel and look vibrantly healthy, happy and eternally radiant.

Deborah Garland
Eternal Radiance Ayurveda
PO Box 4144
Scottsdale, AZ 85261
deb@eternalra.com

www.ingramcontent.com/pod-product-compliance
Lightning Source LLC
Chambersburg PA
CBHW080328270326
41927CB00014B/3138